THE
Buena Salud®
GUIDE TO
ARTHRITIS
AND
YOUR LIFE

Other Books by Jane L. Delgado, Ph.D., M.S.

The Buena Salud® *Guide to Overcoming Depression
and Enjoying Life*

The Buena Salud® *Guide for a Healthy Heart*

The Buena Salud® *Guide to Diabetes and Your Life*

The Latina Guide to Health: Consejos *and Caring Answers*

(all available in English and Spanish)

THE
Buena Salud®
GUIDE TO
ARTHRITIS
AND
YOUR LIFE

JANE L. DELGADO, PH.D., M.S.

Foreword by Dr. John H. Klippel, President and CEO,
Arthritis Foundation

WILLIAM MORROW

An Imprint of HarperCollins*Publishers*

Buena Salud® is a registered trademark of Jane L. Delgado.

THE *BUENA SALUD*® GUIDE TO ARTHRITIS AND YOUR LIFE. Copyright © 2012 by Jane L. Delgado. All rights reserved. Printed in the United States of America. No part of this book may be used or reproduced in any manner whatsoever without written permission except in the case of brief quotations embodied in critical articles and reviews. For information address HarperCollins Publishers, 10 East 53rd Street, New York, NY 10022.

HarperCollins books may be purchased for educational, business, or sales promotional use. For information please write: Special Markets Department, HarperCollins Publishers, 10 East 53rd Street, New York, NY 10022.

FIRST EDITION

Library of Congress Cataloging-in-Publication Data has been applied for.

ISBN 978-0-06-219592-0

12 13 14 15 16 DIX/RRD 10 9 8 7 6 5 4 3 2 1

∿ Contents

CONTENTS

The *Buena Salud*® Series

The mission of the National Alliance for Hispanic Health (the Alliance) is to improve the health of Hispanic communities and work with others to secure health for all. This has been a major challenge because although one out of every six people in the United States is Hispanic, too often research, analysis, and recommendations do not address Hispanic lives. As information emerges about Hispanic health, it is clear that to achieve the best health outcomes for all, we need a different approach to health care in our communities. Besides providing the best health information, we need to create a new way to think about health that blends the strengths of the Hispanic community with the latest medical and technological advances.

The *Buena Salud*® series is designed to make that happen. Each book identifies the key factors that define a health concern, the changes that each of us needs to consider making for ourselves and our family, the most up-to-date information to live healthier lives, and the tools that we need to make that possible.

The challenge is to sort through the daily onslaught of health-related information and recognize that many of the changes we need to make to improve our health we cannot do alone. Our sense of family and responsibility to our family is one of the great strengths in our community, and it is key to improving the health system. Nevertheless, to do so we all need to work together. Whether it is an uncle, a brother, a sister, or a *comadre*, we have to help each other become as healthy as possible. This series is for you because there is so much that you can do to improve your own health and the health of others.

We are at a critical moment when we can make all of our lives better. The promise of science is before us, and we must use every bit of information to care for our bodies, minds, and spirits. Through the *Buena Salud*® series, we want to be your partner in making it happen.

ᔕ Foreword

Taking a walk. Twisting the top off a bottle of aspirin. Gripping a pen. Playing with your children or grandchildren. These are the activities of life many of us take for granted. But for more than 50 million people with arthritis, many of the tasks and joys of daily life can be a challenge.

Those challenges can be made easier. Understanding the challenges and changes arthritis brings can help us live our lives to the fullest. That's why *The* Buena Salud® *Guide to Arthritis and Your Life* deserves a place in every American household. It offers hope.

It is a must-read guide to preventing, managing, and living a full and healthy life with arthritis. Dr. Jane Delgado offers caring advice filled with common sense and empathy. This is the kind of advice you would expect from a best friend, except this best friend also happens to be one of our nation's leading health experts.

In this volume of her *Buena Salud®* Guide series, Dr. Delgado reminds us all that when it comes to arthritis, movement is the best medicine. She walks the reader through the most common questions people have about arthritis, a disease that can strike people of all ages and is the leading cause of disability in our nation.

With her 10-Point Program for Health and Wellness, Dr. Delgado offers us all steps we can take and help our loved ones to take for better health. She helps readers understand how arthritis can affect other chronic conditions, your stress and mood, and your relationships.

Dr. Delgado knows that some of the best advice on arthritis comes from those who have already walked in your shoes. She offers the wisdom of the real-life stories of those living with arthritis and their loved ones. Reading the stories is an inspiration. You know you are not alone in your journey to good health and that there are practical solutions to making every aspect of your life easier and better.

Those stories are woven together with the latest in science and medicine. Dr. Delgado demystifies what can be a confusing diagnosis with easy-to-follow descriptions of conditions, diagnostic terms, and treatments. She offers tools for being an advocate for your, or a loved one's, best health by providing questions to ask your health provider, tools for tracking your health status, and guides to medication.

Dr. Delgado also identifies websites and helplines for more information that you can trust. The best sources for information, finding a health provider, local support groups, help with the cost of care, and other critical issues are all here and organized in an easy-to-use format. This is a book you will refer to over and over again.

The Buena Salud® *Guide to Arthritis and Your Life* is an indispensable road map for those with arthritis and their loved ones to living their best lives.

DR. JOHN H. KLIPPEL
PRESIDENT AND CEO
ARTHRITIS FOUNDATION

ᔡ Introduction

I know when my neck started to hurt. Years ago I
had been working long hours and to save time I
decided to carry all of my supplies in two bags—
one on each shoulder. Then one day as I was
running from one job to the next I felt excruciating
pain and that was the start of this situation. It
seems like I have always had this pain. —Roberto

Arthritis is one of the conditions that is taken for granted
because it does not kill you. Too often the focus is on
diseases that kill us rather than conditions that can
compromise how we live. When arthritis is ignored, the consequences will be negative on many aspects of our lives. If you or
someone you know has arthritis, you need to know what you
can do to make life easier.

For many people the first sign of arthritis starts with pain in
one knee. For others the pain is in the hip, hands, wrist, or the
back of the neck. What you feel is a sharp pain in one of your
joints.

Usually you can find an explanation for the pain you feel—
you injured yourself or you did too much of some activity. In
most instances you take care of the pain by resting and taking a couple of pills you can buy without a prescription. You
tell yourself that the pain is nothing or that maybe you have a
touch of arthritis. You shrug your shoulders and keep on going.

But pain is a symptom that should signal that something
might be more complicated than it appears. This is especially

true as that touch of self-diagnosed arthritis you downplay becomes harder to ignore. As the pain and discomfort become intense or occur more often, you may feel that you do not have to see your health care provider because you assume it is just arthritis.

In many ways, however, believing you have arthritis is like knowing you have a fever. While it is good to know when your temperature is above normal, what you really need to know is what made your temperature go up.

That is why you need to see your health care provider to determine what condition is causing the pain and inflammation in your joints. There are nearly 100 conditions that can cause arthritis and knowing which one you have is essential. An accurate diagnosis will ensure that you receive the treatment that is best for you.

It is interesting the response I get when someone has told me he has arthritis and I ask him what type of arthritis he has. He looks at me perplexed because he believes that saying that he has arthritis should be enough information to understand his situation.

Of great concern is that most people think the pain and discomfort of arthritis is something that happens as a result of getting older. The thought that usually follows is that it is a condition you have to accept and just live with. In other words, that there is nothing you can do to prevent it or get rid of it.

Arthritis is not just a result of getting older; there are children who have arthritis. According to the Centers for Disease Control and Prevention (CDC), in the United States there are nearly 50 million people, or one in five adults, who have been diagnosed with arthritis by their health care provider, as well as approximately 300,000 children who have arthritis. The proportion of non-Hispanic whites, African-Americans, and Hispanics with arthritis is about the same. The number of Hispanics with arthritis may be underrepresented because fewer have access to health care providers.

Hispanics, however, are twice as likely as non-Hispanic whites to report severe joint pain and work limitations because of their arthritis. We have very limited information on how many people in the United States have specific conditions that produce arthritis. We do know that 28 percent of people over 45 years old and 45 percent of people over 65 have osteoarthritis of the knee. Unfortunately, based on statistics like this, it is easy to wrongly assume that just being older produces arthritis. In fact, arthritis is a disease that in most instances starts when you are younger and gets worse over time. This is why it is considered a chronic degenerative disease. As noted previously, arthritis also occurs in children.

This book is intended to help you understand the complexities of arthritis, inform you about key topics, and provide you with the tools to help you improve how you handle arthritis. You have to remember that you are not alone in trying to make life better. Throughout this book you will hear the voices of people who live with arthritis. The doubts and challenges that they share should encourage you to move forward.

As part of the *Buena Salud*® series, my goal is to provide information in a way that is relevant to you. Like a *tía* who adores you and has wisdom and science to share, these books are in a familiar format. Part One focuses on the basic information you need to know. This ranges from what a joint is to a discussion of the immune system so that you understand some of the basics about arthritis. This is especially helpful when you visit your health care provider. Part Two provides information on the major conditions that cause arthritis and the latest research on all those treatments you hear about. This also includes differentiating which treatments are a waste of your money and time from those that have proven to be more effective options. Part Three gives you the resources you need to organize your life to minimize the impact of arthritis. It includes the best online sources for information about the management of arthritis and tools for maintaining a healthy lifestyle.

Too many of us believe that the best thing to do for pain in our joints is to ignore it. This book tells you the simple steps you can take to reduce pain, improve your ability to move, and make your life better. Keep in mind that arthritis is a symptom of many conditions, and when you do the best you can to manage it, you will be able to enjoy your life even more. But most of all I want to give you a message of hope. There is much that you can do now that will help you live with arthritis, and there is even more to look forward to with the new scientific discoveries in the field of arthritis.

Part One

UNDERSTANDING ARTHRITIS

About your life

At church I look and wonder how everyone else, even some women who I know are much older than I am, are able to kneel. I certainly cannot do that; the pain would be too great. I can't remember when kneeling became such a problem for me. I don't know when it all changed. There was no single event. I guess that what was a small pain got worse over time, and I ignored the changes. And now, because of my neglect, I cannot even kneel. —Loretta

Just a few weeks ago, I got together with some of the other guys I know to watch a football game. The television had to be moved, and I was the only one who could move it as they all had arthritis from old injuries. Is that what happens to everyone? —Alonso

What do you do when you have pain, or when you feel very tired? Too many of us are so focused on the immediate demands of daily life that we ignore that our body is trying to tell us something is wrong. We assume that pain or fatigue is something that will eventually go away. And in some cases it might, but in others it just continues until one day we can barely move.

My mother was one of those people who had pain but, no matter what, she would go to work and do whatever she had to do to get through the day. It didn't matter whether she had such pain in her neck that it would make her face feel numb or whether her fingers were so swollen she could not grip the tools she needed for her job, her focus was on getting her job done. She was the sole supporter of the family, and she knew all too well that others would eagerly take her spot on the factory floor. Pain was something she simply learned to live with.

Aguantar, or to endure difficulties without complaining, was the theme that was woven through her daily experience. In an odd way, the pain became an unwanted constant companion that tinted her every thought and movement. After a while the pain was so familiar that her tendency was to forget about it. Even when she saw her health care provider the pain was shuffled to the back of her health priorities. But pain is your body talking to you, and you have to learn to listen to it.

Too often our sense of obligation to our responsibilities and to our work makes it difficult to take time off; some of us do not even have the option of taking sick leave to heal ourselves. As a result, our strong work ethic becomes a factor in our deteriorating health. Moreover, our values about endurance and caring for family can create barriers to seeking help.

We need to put aside all those beliefs that make it difficult to seek help. Whether it is the feminine or masculine concept of "being strong"—*aguantando* or *machismo*—or the desire to be a superwoman or a superman, we need to put that aside and do something about the pain we feel.

We have to care for ourselves as well as we care for others. What we should do is treat ourselves the way we would treat someone in our family who had pain that made it difficult to move and that seemed to get worse with time. We need to accept that taking care of ourselves is not only how we take care of our families but also a demonstration of a deeper sense of strength.

We should not let pain and discomfort frame our life. As a first step, we need to have some idea of what may be happening to our body and what we can do to reduce, if not eliminate, the pain to maintain our level of activity. We want to be able to live and take care of our own situation, but to do so, we need to know the facts that are available to us today.

What is arthritis?

When someone says she has arthritis she usually means that she has pain, inflammation, and stiffness in one or more of her joints. In the past a person might have said that she had rheumatism. Regardless of what you call the discomfort you experience, it is important to know that it could be a sign of one of many conditions. Be certain that although your friend or *tía* is very wise, only your health care provider can tell you what actual condition you have. And even for your health care provider, it may be difficult to diagnose quickly because there are more than 100 conditions that are designated as rheumatic diseases. Also there is no single test that will tell your health care provider instantly which one you have.

> I've had pains in all my joints since I was little.
> My parents were told that I had rheumatism
> and that there was little that they could do for
> me. —Aurora

It is not surprising that there is much confusion when we talk among ourselves about arthritis. It seems that the word *arthritis* has many meanings and uses.

The word *arthritis* comes from ancient Greek. "Arthro" is a prefix that means "joint," and "itis" is a suffix that means "inflammation." You are told you have arthritis when you have inflammation in one or more of your joints (the juncture where two or more bones meet).

Inflammation (indicated by redness, swelling, pain, often warm to the touch) is a response to an injury and is the way our immune system usually protects us. When the inflammation lasts too long, however, it can damage tissue and that causes pain. This is why arthritis is a symptom rather than a disease itself.

The everyday use of the word *arthritis* covers an assortment of different diseases that are clustered under conditions or diseases that affect the joints or connective tissue. There are more than 100 arthritic conditions, which may affect one or more joints, tendons (connections between bone and a muscle), or ligaments (fibrous collagenlike tissue that connects bone to another bone). Joints are made up of ligaments, bones, muscles, and connective tissues that connect many internal parts.

Osteoarthritis is the most common arthritic condition and is usually caused by the wearing down of cartilage (the lining that covers the bone) and bone in a joint. Other rheumatic conditions include autoimmune diseases, which occur when the immune system, instead of protecting the body, mistakes a part of the body for a disease-causing contaminant and attacks it. Rheumatoid arthritis is the most common of the autoimmune diseases that cause arthritis. Some of the other types of rheumatic diseases are (in alphabetical order): ankylosing spondylitis, complex regional pain syndrome, dermatomyositis, fibromyalgia, gout, juvenile idiopathic arthritis, lupus (systemic lupus erythematosus, or SLE), polymyalgia rheumatica, polymyositis, rheumatoid arthritis, and scleroderma.

To add to the confusion the terms *arthritis* and *rheumatic conditions* are sometimes used interchangeably. Maybe the best place to begin is by understanding some of the basics about joints and our immune system.

Know your joints

A joint is where two or more bones come together. There are different types of joints. Some joints are fixed and do not move. For example, the bones in your skull come together but do not move. Most joints, however, are meant to help you move.

When you refer to a joint, you are talking about many parts. These may include the bone, cartilage (which is at the end of the bone and covers it), muscles, ligaments, synovium (the lining of the joint that releases synovial fluid, which acts as a lubricant for the joint), and an area of dense collagen that covers the entire joint (joint capsule). Synovial fluid reduces the friction between the bones in the joint.

Your knees, hips, shoulders, elbows, and neck have joints. You also have joints in your hands and feet. These joints make it possible for your bones to move without pain because at the end of the bone is cartilage, which acts as a cushion. These joints have two functions: (1) to allow for movement between the bones, and (2) to absorb impact from your movement or repetitive motions. The cartilage prevents the bones from grinding against each other. When your joints work well, you are able to stay active and independent.

A key component of the joint is the cartilage. The cartilage is made up of mostly water (65 to 80 percent) and collagen (which helps strengthen the joint), proteoglycans (which allow for flexing and shock absorption), and chrondrocytes (which produce cartilage and also release an enzyme that destroys collagen). Each of these substances has a special role to make sure that the joint works well. Research is ongoing to develop more effective treatment for damaged cartilage.

Sometimes a joint can become damaged. This damage may occur as a result of injury, by additional stress caused by excess weight, from work that has repetitive movement or requires heavy physical effort, by physical activity done in an unhealthy way, or by some other condition. When a joint is damaged, the bones grind against each other. This causes the pain and inflammation called *arthritis,* and this can produce more loss of bone and cartilage. At other times, the inflammation is caused by a malfunctioning of the immune system.

About your immune system

Your immune system is the warrior within you that fights off disease. Like a personal bodyguard, the immune system carefully monitors every part of your body to destroy all that may be harmful to you. The immune system is located throughout the body in different places: the tonsils and adenoids, the lymph nodes in the throat and the attached lymphatic vessels, the thymus (which is in the middle of the chest), the lymph nodes in the armpits, the spleen (located on your left side, just about where the elbow touches), the appendix (on your right side, halfway between the elbow and wrist), Peyer's patch (to the left of the belly button), lymph nodes and lymphatic vessels in the inner leg area, and the bone marrow throughout the body. All of these sites work to keep you healthy.

Inflammation is a signal that your immune system is working to protect you from infection, such as a virus, bacteria, or some other chemical that is outside of your body. In this instance, inflammation is a good and natural response. When inflammation lasts too long, then you can have problems.

Sometimes your immune system malfunctions and works too little or too much. When your immune system is not very active, you have an immunodeficiency. This means that your immune system does not protect you and is asleep on the job. At other times the immune system is too aggressive and, instead of protecting you, mistakenly attacks you. The diseases that result are called autoimmune diseases. You have an auto-immune disorder when the immune system causes inflammation, even though nothing is attacking you.

The processes that keep your immune system working properly are controlled by many factors. One of these factors are cytokines, a type of molecule that tells your cells what to do. These molecules tell the immune system when to increase or decrease inflammation, as well as when to make more cells available that reabsorb bone. In most instances, inflammation is a good response.

Today, some of the medicines available to treat arthritis usually work either to reduce the activity of certain molecules and cells that increase inflammation (anti-inflammatory) or to suppress the immune system. Since arthritis has so many aspects, your care will be in the hands of a variety of health care providers. Some of these different health care providers are described in the next chapter.

About your health care providers

Arthritis is usually experienced as pain, stiffness, or difficulty doing physical tasks you could easily do before. If you suffer from any of these symptoms, you should see your health care provider. This is especially important for Hispanics, who are more likely to experience missed workdays and disability related to their arthritis and, at the same time, are the group least likely to see a health care provider. Discussing symptoms with your health care provider as soon as you feel them is important, so that diagnosis can be made early and a treatment plan developed to maximize your movement and limit pain.

If you do not have a regular source of health care, it would be good to identify one. A health care professional with a specialty in internal medicine or a gerontologist (a specialist in medicine for older persons) may be a good place to start. For children, you should see a pediatrician, who may in turn refer you to another specialist.

Based on the preliminary assessment of your joints and the results of any additional tests, if your health care provider believes that you have an autoimmune disease, you may be referred to a rheumatologist or a clinical immunologist. A rheumatologist is a health care provider who focuses on rheumatic or musculoskeletal conditions. You may also be referred to a clinical immunologist, who treats disorders of the immune system.

In addition to a rheumatologist or a clinical immunologist, there are also a variety of different health professionals for spe-cific services. Some of these are listed below, in alphabetical order, followed by a short description:

- **Acupuncturist (licensed therapist):** a health professional who inserts hair-thin needles into specific body points to decrease pain and improve health and well-being.
- **Chiropractor:** a health professional who uses an alternative medical system that treats health problems with a hands-on therapy called spinal manipulation or adjustment.
- **Massage therapist:** a health professional who manipulates the muscles and soft tissues of your body.
- **Nephrologist:** a health care professional who specializes in the care of kidneys.
- **Nurse/nurse practitioner:** a health care professional who assists the physician in caring for your arthritis.
- **Occupational therapist:** a health professional who works with you to develop ways for you to move so that you can continue in your current occupation.
- **Orthopedic surgeon:** a surgeon who specializes in the treatment and surgery of bone and joint diseases.
- **Physiatrists (rehabilitation specialists):** a health professional who helps you maximize your activity within the limitations of your joint problem.
- **Physical therapist:** a health professional who assesses your range of motion and then works with you to implement a plan to increase the painless movement of your joints.

- **Psychologist:** a health professional who focuses on the treatment of psychological issues, including depression.
- **Social worker:** a professional who helps you adjust to the social challenges you may encounter, including disability, unemployment, and home health care.

You will work with your team of health care providers to develop a treatment plan that will be aimed at helping you maintain as much mobility as possible, stabilize the progression of your condition, and reduce pain. What you will need to do requires more than just visiting different health professionals. To ensure the success of your treatment plan, it is essential for you to rethink much of what you do so that your actions are consistent with the good health you want to enjoy.

Life changes to consider: things to do and things to avoid

In order to manage your arthritis you need to make a commitment to strengthen key parts of your life. The 10-Point Program for Health and Wellness is designed to support you as you take steps to be healthy and happy. It is based on the emerging science that shows there is no single action that is the magic bullet for health. In fact, what the data show are that many factors lead to health and wellness. Although the letters TLC usually are shorthand for tender loving care, as we move forward in our life they also represent therapeutic lifestyle changes (TLC). Taking both meanings together the message is simply that we have to care for ourselves as well as we care for others. We need to recognize that there are a variety of steps to take to feel good and be healthy.

That is why the elements that make up the 10-Point Program are classified as either core items or magnifiers. Core items—#1 through #4—are your "must-do items." As you read the following sections, you will learn the latest techniques for creating and maintaining positive behaviors in these areas. Although your health care provider may have made suggestions to you about what you should do, you already know what you need to do. The challenge is to make the adjustments in your life so you can do them.

Magnifiers are items #5 through #10. These take the benefits of your core activities and supercharge them. When you do them, they boost the benefits of your core actions (#1 through #4), and when you do not do them, that may diminish the impact of your core efforts.

Once you know the condition that is causing your arthritis, you will have to think about these 10 Points and how to tailor them to your situation. It may mean that you have to eat different foods or rethink your exercise program. There are activities that you may have liked to do that you now have to reconsider, and others that you have never tried that you now have to incorporate into your life. You need to re-create an environment that supports you in your efforts to live a life that is as healthy as possible. This may not be easy to do when we have to deal with pain and discomfort. We tend to do what is familiar and easy even when it is not good for us.

The challenge is knowing how to reorganize your life. A good place to start is to do a quick self-assessment of what you are doing. There are no right or wrong answers as this is information to help you understand your lifestyle.

Look at the following questions, then think about what it means for a statement to be true, and honestly assess whether the statement is true for you. A "True" response does not mean that you always do something, but rather that you do it at least 95 percent of the time, or, put another way, at least 19 out of 20 times.

Look at your answers as information to help you plan what you can do to live a healthier life. If you have some items that are "True," those are items for celebration. That does not mean

1. I eat and drink for a healthy body. ☐True ☐False

2. I exercise at least 5 times a week. ☐True ☐False

3. I take all my medications. ☐True ☐False

4. I have a regular source of
   health care. ☐True ☐False

5. I stay away from smoke and other
   toxic substances. ☐True ☐False

6. I get enough sleep. ☐True ☐False

7. I have healthy relationships. ☐True ☐False

8. I keep a journal of my health. ☐True ☐False

9. I cherish my spiritual life. ☐True ☐False

10. I know how to listen to my body. ☐True ☐False

that you forget about them because instead you may want to fine-tune these items to maximize their impact.

The opportunity and the challenge are defined by those items that you indicated are "False." For the most part, the fact that these are important steps for health and wellness is not new. These 10 statements are basic to the understanding of what is good to do. The challenge is to figure out for each statement what adjustments you need to make in your life so that the statement is true for you.

After you read the following sections, you have to decide what are the steps that you need to take. Your plan should be one that will work for you. While some people will want to work on all the "False" responses at once, most people will target only a few elements. Ideally perhaps you should start with the core items, but actually the best place to start is wherever you will be most motivated to make the changes you need to make. The 10-Point Program is designed for you because you choose where to start and what to do. The hard work is to have the program become embedded in your life; it is about making life changes and not just a stopgap program. After all, it is your life that you want to enjoy.

1. EAT AND DRINK FOR A HEALTHY BODY

IT IS IMPORTANT TO EAT A BALANCED DIET AND TO GET ENOUGH calcium and vitamin D to keep your bones strong. Most of the time I tell people not to focus on their weight and just focus on being healthy. When it comes to pain and inflammation of the joints, the message is different because there is a close link between the severity of symptoms and excess weight. This makes sense because the less weight a joint has to carry the less stress on the hip and knee joints. At a fundamental level excess weight increases the mechanical stress on the joints. And more stress results in more pain.

There is also a strong relationship between having excess weight and having limitations in daily activities. For example, while people of all sizes may have osteoarthritis, people who are overweight double their risk of osteoarthritis while those who are obese quadruple their risk. That is why in 2011 the CDC reported that the rate at which arthritis occurred (prevalence) was 29.6 percent for people who are obese, 19.8 percent for people who are overweight, and 16.9 percent for people who were normal or underweight.

The good news is that you can start by losing just a few pounds. You do not have to have a huge weight loss for your joints to enjoy some benefit. In fact, modest weight loss of 10 to 12 pounds or 5 percent of your body weight has been shown to reduce pain symptoms. The benefits of maintaining a healthier weight go beyond the reduction of pain in your joints. When adults with osteoarthritis who have excess weight do lose weight, they may also reduce the likelihood of dying early by nearly 50 percent.

To lose weight is challenging; and to maintain that weight loss is even more difficult because often people who have been diagnosed with arthritis may have to temper their physical activity. According to the CDC, the process of weight loss and maintenance of a healthy weight are even more complex for people with arthritis since they may have real limitations in their physical activity. What this means is that new methods for weight loss and the maintenance of that loss need to be developed that take into account what a person can physically do as well as what resources are available to them to support these efforts. For example, while swimming is a good activity on many fronts, few people have ongoing access to places where they can swim. Activities that are joint-friendly and resource-neutral need to be identified.

Given these limitations, a good place to begin is to restart our relationship with food. We have to think of eating not as something we do on some set schedule but rather as an aspect of our life that needs to be updated to meet the needs of our joints. Try to think about yourself and understand the who, what, where, when, and why of eating. Let's take these one at a time and see how they should help you rethink how you eat.

Who. It is important to eat your meals with people who will support your healthy eating habits. The people who sit down with you to eat should respect your goal of eating healthy. At the same time you have to recognize that you are not the food police; others may choose to eat in a way that is unhealthy.

What. There was a recent study that found that most weight gain could be attributed to eating French fries, chips, and sweetened drinks. This is not a surprise. Too often what we eat, whether at home or in restaurants, is determined by what is available quickly and easily. We need to think about food and how our body will use it.

Where. All the data point to the importance of eating at home or taking home-cooked meals with you to eat at work. It may be easier to eat at a quick-serve or fast-food restaurant, but you have more control over what you eat and how much you eat when you eat at home.

When. While you may be in a rush in the morning, eating breakfast is a good way to start the day. Additionally for most people, it is best not to eat too late. For everyone it is best to eat at regular times. You have to eat when you want to eat and not just because everyone else wants to eat. The best practice is to eat small, frequent meals when you want to eat and stop when you are full.

Why. If you eat because you feel sad or angry or just because the food is there, then you need to stop and think. You have to remind yourself that you eat because you need to eat healthy food to stay healthy.

To help you lose weight you also need to be aware of the 3Ps of healthy eating: pleasure, portion, and process.

Pleasure

Think about what you are eating and how you are eating, while enjoying the flavors, smells, textures, and nutritional value of the foods you are consuming. It is not good to eat without thinking about your food. If you find you are finished eating before everyone else, then you are eating too fast. To have a healthy weight you need to consider more than just the calories; you also need to think about how satisfying the food is. If you eat without thinking, then you will not be giving your body the fuel it needs to function well and you will not be as healthy or as satisfied as you could be.

Along similar lines we drink to replenish our bodies that are mostly water, and this is why it is important to drink what is good for us. Drinks that dehydrate us work against our health, and drinking alcohol adds calories that provide no health benefit. In fact, too much alcohol can lead to *alcohol abuse* (when people drink to excess, but do not have a physical addiction) or *alcoholism* (when people have physical signs of addiction). In general, those at risk for alcoholism are:

- Men who have 15 or more drinks a week.
- Women who have 12 or more drinks a week.
- Men or women who have 5 or more drinks per occasion at least once a week.

Keep in mind that one drink is a 12-ounce bottle of beer, a 5-ounce glass of wine, or a 1½-ounce shot of hard liquor. Sometimes, when you order a "mixed drink," there are three or four different shots in one glass. So your one glass may actually be the equivalent of two or three drinks. When it comes to alcohol, you have to be honest about what you are drinking.

Portion
The portion you serve yourself should be whatever is the right amount for you. Too often the concept of portion has been driven by "bigger is better," when in fact portions should be "tailor-made." In other words, what is a good portion for a younger person who is physically active is too large a portion for someone who is older and is more sedentary.

The portions served at many restaurants are often too large. Nevertheless, too often you may feel compelled to eat all of this food because you or someone else paid for it. Even when you buy prepared foods, it is important to read the portion size and the nutritional information that is on the label. I remember buying a package that had three pieces of baked banana. You can imagine my surprise when I read that the nutritional information was per serving and that each package contained four servings. The only way that the three bananas would come to four portions would be if you cut a quarter off each banana. The nutritional information was helpful, but the packaging to me was deceptive.

Determining what is a proper portion for you needs to be based on several factors:

1. *As you get older your metabolism tends to slow down, so you should eat less.* While it may be true

that when you were younger you ate a lot more and now you eat less, the reality is that to lose weight you may have to decrease even more what you eat.

2. *There is a strong relationship between your level of physical activity and your weight goals.* When you are more physically active, you will need to increase your portions to maintain your weight or eat the same amount or less if you want to lose weight. When you are less physically active, you will need to decrease your portions to maintain your weight and you will have to decrease them even more to lose weight.

3. *Just because it is served does not mean you have to eat it all.* A good strategy is to eat half of the food on your plate and save the rest for a future lunch or dinner. Think of it as a 2-for-1 deal! As for dessert, in most instances consider it to be something to be shared. If you are at a birthday party, you do not have to say, "No, thank you," or "I can't eat cake." Instead you might say, "Let me have a sliver," and then only eat a bite. Most important of all, think of that bite you take as your first and last bite. Enjoy it.

4. *You have to be honest about what is the right-sized portion for you.* We are not all the same size, and the portion that someone else takes may be the wrong size for you. And remember that just because it is served, was expensive, was made with love just for you, or whatever emotional strings are played does not mean that you have to eat it all.

If the portion you eat is the right amount for you, then you will maintain your weight; if you eat slightly less, you will lose weight; and if you eat more than your body needs, your body may store it in places you would rather it not.

Being aware of the size of portions is important, and just as critical is recognizing when you are actually full as opposed to being stuffed. Think of "full" as being satiated and "stuffed" as being packed like a sausage. It is good to be satiated, but unhealthy to be stuffed. The goal is to know the difference.

Keep in mind that your stomach and your digestive system can hold a lot of food, so it is not an issue of capacity. Think of what happens to the insides of people who enter eating contests. Some of them eat more than 50 hot dogs in less than 10 minutes. The challenge for you is to know when you have had enough and then to stop. In most instances your capacity to consume food is greater than what is healthy for you. Portion control is about knowing what is right for you; this means you stop eating when you know you have consumed enough nutrition.

Process
We now know that calories are only part of the story, albeit an important part of the story. Science is starting to reveal that more processed foods tend to be less filling or satisfying. They may even stimulate our cravings, which makes it harder to feel that we have had enough. It is often not clear what part of the processing is most unhealthy, but that is not as important as knowing that you have to eat fewer processed foods.

People with some conditions, especially gout, have to further modify what they eat in very specific ways. For most of us, the simplest way to deal with foods that are processed is to avoid them. The healthiest way is to *eat brown* (brown rice, whole-wheat pasta, whole-grain breads, and, yes, the occasional dark chocolate), *eat a variety of what is colorful* (eating what is green, yellow, red, and orange means enjoying an assortment of vegetables and fruits, such as kale, bananas, tomatoes, avocados, chili peppers, sweet potatoes, beans, and greens), *avoid white* (sugar, salt, fat, white bread, white rice, and white potatoes), and add a little bit of meat, chicken, or fish.

Eating healthy is about enjoying what we eat because it is good for us.

2. EXERCISE FOR LIFE

IN ORDER TO BE HEALTHY, WE HAVE TO MOVE AROUND MORE. Research has shown that people who sit for too long during the day are more likely to die prematurely. We all know that movement is good, but how do you temper that with the reality that joint pain, which defines arthritis, can make movement painful? The objective is to find the movement you can do and do that as frequently as possible for as long as you can. Research shows that increasing the strength around your joint can lessen your joint pain. For example, walking is a wonderful way to get movement into your life.

According to the Physical Activity Guidelines for Americans, the weekly goals for adults are at least:

- 150 minutes of moderate-intensity aerobic activity
  (brisk walking) and muscle strengthening 2 or
  more days that works all the major muscle groups
  (legs, hips, back, abdomen, chest, shoulders,
  and arms); or
- 75 minutes of vigorous-intensity aerobic activity
  (jogging or running) and muscle strengthening
  2 or more days that works all the major muscle
  groups (legs, hips, back, abdomen, chest, shoulders,
  and arms); or
- A combination of moderate and vigorous aerobic
  activity and muscle strengthening 2 or more
  days that works all the major muscle groups
  (legs, hips, back, abdomen, chest, shoulders,
  and arms).

Applying these guidelines to the daily activity of someone who may have limitations requires creativity and thinking of physical activity in a new way. Begin by realizing that if you add something extra to your day, that single action in and of itself is more than you were doing before. And more movement is good.

If more is good, then smart movement is even better. This means that you already have a good sense of what you can and cannot do. If you are in pain, you cannot exercise that area but you may be able to do some other activity. For example, when you have knee pain, perhaps you can focus on your upper body or focus on more stretching and relaxation type of movements. You may even want to try something new like tai chi. Research has indicated that tai chi exercise may improve your quality of life, your mood, and even your feelings about being able to do exercise. You can find resources to help you make movement a daily part of your life on pages 107–9.

The best exercise program is the one you will follow. So in order to do more and do it in a smart way, here are some things for you to remember.

1. **Check what you can do.** Talk to your health care provider about any recommendations that he or she may have about what you should or should not do.

2. **Start where you are.** You want to start your plan at the stage you are now in terms of physical activity and exertion. Do not start where you left off the last time you exercised, or base your start level at what you remember you could do at another point in your life. Your abilities change over time, and you need to be realistic about what you can and cannot do.

3. **Begin slowly.** You do not want to overdo it, because if you do, it is likely you will injure yourself. If your goal is to walk one mile, start by walking one block; if you want to be able to touch your toes, start by touching your knees. Slow progress is the best because it gives you the opportunity to build up your ability over time.

4. **Avoid pain.** It is not good to push through the pain or to "feel the burn." When you do that, you end up injuring yourself. If it hurts to stand then do exercises sitting. You can do a lot of movement from a sitting position.

When I went to see the orthopedist he told me
I had arthritis in my knee. He suggested that I
take some over-the-counter ibuprofen. Much to
my surprise, he also said I needed to stretch my
calves and thighs because they were too tight
from sitting all day. It seems that the arthritis in
my knee is aggravated when I do not stretch the
other muscles around it. So now every morning
before I get out of bed, I do 20 leg lifts with
each leg. And it actually helps. —Marcos

5. **Total exercises.** Exercises are for your heart, your
   bones (they are alive too), your joints, and your
   muscles. All these parts work together to keep
   you healthy and active. Unfortunately, there is no
   single exercise that is perfect for every person and
   every condition. You have to find aerobic exercises
   that are good for your heart, strengthening
   exercises such as weight-bearing activities that you
   can do, and activities that increase your flexibility
   so you can move with ease. Both men and women
   need these three types of exercises. Stretching is
   essential to maintaining your flexibility. There is
   no need for fancy equipment or expensive health
   clubs. Elastic bands are low-cost items that you can
   use to help you stretch. You can even use towels.
   The key is to begin gently and to stretch. If you do
   not know what exercise is good for arthritis, ask
   your health care provider.

6. **No comparisons.** Do not compare yourself to
   anyone else you know or watch or see. You need

to focus on the goals that you set for yourself. This will keep you motivated. When you see someone else doing some activity, you only know what you see and not all the preparation that may have led up to that point. You are you, and the fact that you have increased your movement is enormous.

7. **No jumping.** The high-impact aerobics that were popular in the 1980s ended up causing many of the injuries that were experienced as people got older. For some people with arthritis, low-impact aerobics (this usually means you keep at least one foot on the ground) provide the level of exercise that is safe for their joints and what they need for their heart. Others may prefer the joint-friendly movements that come with swimming, bicycling, tai chi, or easy yoga.

8. **Feet are key.** Wear shock-absorbing shoes and in some cases you may also want to add weight-dampening inserts. These help to make movement easier and less painful.

9. **Know when to stop.** Although you may have a plan that you are following diligently on some days, you may need to give yourself a rest. The point of exercise is not to keep going until exhaustion or injury, but rather to establish a pattern that builds your strength, flexibility, and endurance.

10. **Be fierce and joyful.** Whatever you do, it has to be something that you enjoy. It is hard to stay with

> any program if you do not like it. Some people
> find making plans to exercise with others keeps
> them on their exercise regimen, while others
> prefer to exercise by themselves. Try to consider
> and explore new activities that do not involve any
> upfront financial investment.

What we know is that for people with osteoarthritis, just walking has positive results. Not only will they be able to walk farther gradually but they will also gradually experience less pain.

3. TAKE YOUR MEDICATIONS (PRESCRIPTION AND OVER-THE-COUNTER)

THE TREATMENT FOR ARTHRITIS USUALLY INVOLVES A COMBINATION of weight loss, exercise, and medications that you will need to follow for the rest of your life. As your condition changes, the medicines you take may also change. To help you keep track and remember when to take your medicines, it is good to set up a routine that is easy to follow. If you live with other people, it is good for them to know your routine so that they can support your efforts to take your medicines. It also helps to keep a list of your medications in an easily accessible place and to know what they look like, when you are supposed to take them, and any special instructions that will help you. Be sure to tell your health care provider all the medicines you are taking, including over-the-counter ones, as well as herbal medicines, supplements, and teas.

When you receive your medicines be sure to read the information on the label and whatever supporting documents are included. If you do not understand the instructions, you need to talk to the pharmacist or to your health care provider. It is better to get clarification than to take your medicines in a way that will not provide the intended outcome.

4. HAVE A REGULAR SOURCE OF HEALTH CARE

HISPANIC MEN AND WOMEN ARE THE PERSONS LEAST LIKELY TO have a regular source of health care. It is something that we have to change because wellness visits are essential to maintaining your health. Regular visits are also key for assessing how well your medication is working and coming up with other recommendations to make you feel better. Depending on the type of arthritis you have you may have one health care provider or a team of health care providers. How often you see your health care provider will be established in a conversation between you and your health care provider so that there can be ongoing monitoring of your condition.

Going to see health care providers means that you also feel comfortable talking to them about how you feel and how you are doing. I have been surprised by the number of people who tell me that sometimes they do not want to see their health care providers because they do not want to tell them how bad they feel. You should feel comfortable talking to your health care provider. This means that you need to feel that your health care provider listens to you and what you are saying. If you feel uncomfortable with your health care provider then you should seriously consider finding a different one.

The older you are, the more likely that in addition to your arthritis you have other health conditions. You need to know that your health care provider focuses on your total health and not on any single condition to the exclusion of the rest of your health.

5. STAY AWAY FROM SMOKE AND OTHER TOXIC SUBSTANCES

WE KNOW THAT PEOPLE WHO SMOKE ARE MORE LIKELY TO GET rheumatoid arthritis. When you smoke, you are exposing every cell in your body to a known harmful substance. Keep in mind that tobacco enters your body whether you smoke (firsthand smoke), someone near you is smoking (secondhand smoke), or even when you can smell cigarette smoke on some object or person or in some room (thirdhand smoke). There are numerous other chemicals that are not good for you to inhale. Many of them are known as volatile organic compounds, or VOCs, and are released by cleaning supplies, pesticides, building materials, paint, new carpeting, copiers and printers, correction fluids, and carbonless copy paper.

The reason that these chemicals are dangerous is related to how your body works. When you breathe, your lungs work to bring fresh oxygen to the red blood cells that then travel throughout your body to nourish every cell. When what you breathe is harmful, then that is what your red blood cells bring to every cell in your body.

For many reasons it is good to reduce exposure to toxic or harmful chemicals. While some of these may not kill you instantly, most of them cause long-term damage that we are only starting to understand. As our ability to measure the presence of these substances increases, we are learning about how minuscule amounts (20 parts per billion or less) can upset our endocrine system and have a negative impact on our immune system.

At the very least if you do smoke, seek help so that you can stop. If someone you know smokes, support his efforts to stop and stay away from him when he is smoking.

6. GET ENOUGH SLEEP

WHILE WE NEED TO EXERCISE AND KEEP ACTIVE, WE ALSO NEED to make sure that we get enough sleep. Too many of us think sleep is something that is a passive activity that has no important function. We think of sleep as something we have to do, but often shortchange ourselves believing that we can always catch up later. And while this may be true to some extent, there are limitations because of the essential role that sleep plays with respect to our overall health.

The research is clear—sleep is necessary for a person's body to work well. When people do not get enough sleep on a regular basis, they diminish themselves. It is not only their ability to focus and their attention span that is not what it should be, but how their body works is compromised. This is because when you sleep your body produces hormones that help to regulate all aspects of your activity.

Much of what we know about sleep is just evolving. There are people who think that if they sleep less and are active that they will lose weight. The data shows just the opposite is true. For most people, sleeping four to five hours will make them gain weight.

How much sleep you need is based on what you as an individual need. While other members of your family may need eight hours of sleep, you may need more or less. Additionally, the amount of sleep you need changes over time. The chart below provides some guidelines as to how much sleep a person needs by age.

RANGE OF SLEEP NEEDS VARIES BY AGE

AGE	HOURS OF SLEEP NEEDED
Up to 2 months	12–18 hours
3–11 months	14–15 hours
12–36 months	12–14 hours
3–5 years old	11–13 hours
5–10 years old	10–11 hours
10–17 years old	8.5–9.25 hours
18 and older	7–9 hours

Source: National Sleep Foundation website

The importance of regular hours of sleep is based on the fact that your body works on a 24-hour cycle.

People who experience the pain of arthritis may have their sleep disturbed. According to research by the Arthritis Foundation in a survey of 900 people with arthritis, 30 percent had difficulty sleeping because of arthritis. The suggestion from the study was that it was essential for those people to improve their sleep. To minimize disruption it is good to schedule your medications so that you have less pain when you are sleeping.

Recent findings suggest that how much light you are exposed to between dusk and when you go to sleep is very important. It seems that the artificial light from screens (televisions, computers, video games, cell phones, etc.), especially in the hour before you go to sleep, disrupts the production of hormones associated with sleep and upsets your circadian rhythms.

Combining the suggestions from the National Sleep Foundation and the Arthritis Foundation, some of the things you can do to improve your sleep are:

- Time your medicines so that you can reduce the pain when you are sleeping.
- Keep a consistent schedule for going to sleep and waking up. It is more disruptive to have different schedules for the weekend and weekday.
- Control the light in your environment. More light wakes you up and less light will make you sleepy.
- Sleep improves when you participate in physical activity on a regular basis.
- Remove stimulation to make a "sleep space" for yourself. This space should not include the distractions of your work, televisions, computers, etc. To create this environment it may be as simple as covering your eyes and using earplugs.
- Make a space next to your bed or right under your bed where you can store what you need to relax. This may mean a pad to write down thoughts or products that you may use in case of pain.

- When it is approaching the time to go to sleep avoid all products with caffeine, including coffee, tea, chocolate, or energy drinks.
- For some people a bedtime ritual is important to putting themselves in a sleep mode. This varies greatly by individual. For some this is accomplished by praying before going to sleep and for others by reading a few pages of a book or magazine.

When you sleep well, you help reduce the symptoms of arthritis. According to the Arthritis Foundation, "A good night's rest can be an integral part of arthritis treatment."

7. MAINTAIN AND NOURISH HEALTHY RELATIONSHIPS

We were all having a nice Sunday brunch together. When the toast Alicia ordered arrived, her husband, Roberto, asked her if she would like him to butter her toast. I thought that it was sweet that he had offered. Later Alicia told me that it was more than sweet. Roberto asked her because he knew she liked her toast buttered and that she was unable to butter it herself. Alicia added, "And he also has to cut my meat." —Melissa

ARTHRITIS IS A CHRONIC CONDITION THAT YOU NEED TO LEARN TO manage. There will be times, however, when you will need the help of those around you. At those times you will have to ask for assistance, and you need to do that in a way that maintains your self-esteem, reduces stress, and is not burdensome to others. This means that we need to have healthy relationships. The key is to work on having relationships in which there is balance and where each person feels valued and is able to contribute to the relationship. Mental wellness and elimination of stress help reduce pain and discomfort and boost our immune system.

The factors below are important components that foster the healthy relationships essential for our overall health.

Self-esteem

It all starts with you. How you perceive yourself is important for the type of relationships you have. If you have either low or overinflated self-esteem, your relationships become distorted and suffer. Healthy self-esteem means that you value yourself for who you are, and you neither say negative things about yourself nor engage in boastfulness. When you have healthy self-esteem, you know that it is okay to ask others for help. This may be hard for some of us to do because we are used to doing everything for ourselves as well as for everyone else. When two people have healthy self-esteem, they both know how to say yes to each other as well as how to say no.

This is very important when you have arthritis since you have to learn that at times it is okay to ask others for help. The challenge is to do this in a way that maintains your self-esteem.

Balance

Healthy relationships are about balance, so that there is an overall balance of give-and-take and neither person feels either abused or overburdened. The mistake that is often made is interpreting "balance" in a healthy relationship as all actions have to be shared on a 50-50 basis. The reality is that no relationship can always hold firm to those numbers because at different times the needs and resources of each person may vary. Sometimes one person has to give 90 percent and at other times the other person has to give 90 percent because the situation is different. The goal is for giving and receiving to be an *average* of 50-50. That is why healthy relationships are about finding the balance so that neither person feels that he or she is being burdened. This is difficult to do and requires that communication be open and honest.

The good news is that doing something with a partner is better than coping by yourself or even just having him or her do something for you. A study funded by the National Institute of Arthritis and Musculoskeletal and Skin Diseases (NIAMS) at Duke University looked at trying to reduce the pain from osteoarthritis. They tried three different interventions: exercise training for the individual with OA, spouse-assisted pain coping skills training, or a combination of both. The results indicated that there were more improvements with the combination of both than could be achieved by either intervention alone.

Rebalancing

> Sara made it clear that the most difficult part of Miguel's arthritis was that he knew he could no longer work. They had been married for decades and had saved money and made plans for the future. But now that Miguel could not work, Sara could not retire as planned. She would have to work for many more years. —Jane

At times when one person is diagnosed with a condition, it changes the formula on which the relationship was constructed.

The challenge is to discuss how this changes the dynamics and whether there is a need to reconfigure the relationship. This will have to be an ongoing process, with adjustments made along the way. It may mean that you have to seek a range of outside help in order to reorganize your life in the least disruptive way. You may also need to seek professional help on a variety of issues.

8. KEEP A HEALTH JOURNAL

LIFE IS VERY BUSY, AND TOO OFTEN IT IS HARD ENOUGH JUST KEEPing track of birthdays and anniversaries. But to have the best health possible, you need to track your health in a systematic way. Health care has changed, and you have to be your own health advocate. That means you have to be well informed about your health and your condition. If you are fortunate enough to have someone who will be a health advocate for you, that is good. Regardless, whether it is for you or someone else, it is good to have a written record. Too often when we rely on our memory alone, the descriptions are not as accurate as they need to be.

As health is increasingly tailored to the individual, you need to supply your health care provider with the best information about how you have been doing. While the implementation of electronic health records is evolving and one day we will reach the point where consumers will be able to add their information to be instantly accessed, we are not there yet. For the foreseeable future you will have to track how you are doing.

Part Three of this book gives you some tools to help you record your information. You can also use apps on your smartphone if you have one to help you keep your information together. The important action is for you to keep a health journal. Good information about you is key to good decision-making by your health care provider.

9. CHERISH YOUR SPIRITUAL LIFE

WE HAVE NO IDEA WHAT THE BIOLOGICAL PATHWAYS ARE BY which a spiritual life works to make us have better health. What the research shows, however, is that it is an important component of our health. This is especially true when faith is rooted in concepts of love and forgiveness.

While there has been some research on the role of religious/ spiritual coping, the conclusion is generally a recommendation for more research. Part of the problem is that it is difficult to define in a consistently measurable way what is meant by faith or spiritual life.

Since prayer has a calming or soothing effect on some people, it is also likely that these positive feelings impact on the immune system and the endocrine system. It may be that for some people a spiritual life taps into these systems in a way that promotes health.

10. LISTEN TO YOUR BODY

WHEN YOU HAVE ARTHRITIS, YOU LEARN TO LISTEN TO YOUR BODY very carefully. The challenge is not just knowing what to do with the information but also actually doing it. Pain is a very clear signal that something is not doing well, and it is a signal that should not be ignored. When you have pain you have to think about (1) how to alleviate it, and (2) what may have brought it on.

Because of the many factors that impact on your feeling good, keeping a health journal may help you identify triggers and learn more about how your medicines work. It may be that when you look at your health in a more objective manner, you may see the relationship between the onset of pain and what you are doing.

MOVING FORWARD

The 10-Point Program is a good starting point because it is a way to conceptualize your life, and especially your arthritis, not as an isolated occurrence but rather something that requires adjustment in several aspects of your life on an ongoing basis. No one can have perfect health, but we can enjoy *buena salud*. This program is to make your life better, and the best time to start is now.

Keep in mind that some days you may not be as focused on wellness as you should be and that is okay as long as the next day you refocus yourself on taking steps to be healthy. Remember moving forward takes time, but the rewards are many.

Part Two

JUST
THE
FACTS

IF YOU (OR SOMEONE YOU KNOW) ARE DIAGNOSED WITH ARTHRITIS, then you need to have as much information as possible so that you can have a better understanding of this condition. Moreover sometimes a person can have more than one condition that is causing arthritis. A person can have both osteoarthritis and rheumatoid arthritis, for instance. This is another reason why it is good to know as much as possible about this condition and to ask questions.

To increase your understanding, this section provides information on the major rheumatic conditions and the different types of treatment that are most commonly prescribed. Keep in mind that in most instances there is no single test that can determine if you have a specific condition. Your diagnosis will be based on all the information that is available and will include a medical history, physical exam, laboratory tests and procedures, and in some cases different types of imaging procedures. Often it will take more than one visit to get an accurate diagnosis of your condition. In addition to your regular blood tests, your health care provider may ask for some of the special arthritis blood tests below:

- **ANA screen (antinuclear antibody screen).**
  People with some diseases that damage connective tissues, especially lupus or some other autoimmune diseases, often produce antinuclear antibodies. Although the information from this test is useful, it can be misleading because some people who do not have these diseases also have the antibody.
- **CCP (cyclic citrullinated peptide antibody, or anti-CCP).** This test helps to determine if a person

is in the early stages of a more aggressive type of rheumatoid arthritis. It is accurate for 70 percent of the people who have this condition.

- **Complement.** Complement is the name given to a group of proteins that protect you from infection. People who have active lupus have low levels of these substances in their blood.
- **Sed rate (erythrocyte sedimentation rate, or ESR).** High rates usually indicate that there is inflammation. Inflammation is seen in many forms of arthritis, such as rheumatoid arthritis, ankylosing spondylitis, lupus, and scleroderma.
- **Rheumatoid factor.** When this factor is found in people who have rheumatoid arthritis, it usually indicates a more aggressive case. While most people with rheumatoid arthritis have this factor, it is also found in people who do not have it or who may have another disease.

In addition to these blood tests your health care provider may want to examine the synovial fluid in your joints to check the white blood cells, microbes, and other particles that may be there. This procedure is called joint aspiration (arthrocentesis). Your health care provider anesthetizes the joint and then, using a thin needle, draws out some of the synovial fluid.

Your diagnosis will help determine what is the best plan of action for you. For most of the rheumatic conditions, there is treatment but no cure. The only exceptions are when there is early diagnosis of infectious arthritis and Lyme disease. The best way to take care of yourself is to stay informed and active.

⌒ Rheumatic conditions

Osteoarthritis (OA)

Q ¿*Qué pasa?*
You have osteoarthritis when after a series of events the cartilage in your joint can no longer serve as a buffer and allow the bones to slide smoothly over one another when you move. Instead what is happening is that the cartilage is falling apart and disintegrating, making the bones grind and wearing them down. As a result, there is inflammation and pain. Over time small pieces of bone may get into the joint area and cause more pain. In some cases there are small deposits of bone around the joints (bone spurs or osteophytes). As the condition worsens, the joint may lose its normal shape.

Osteoarthritis is the most common rheumatic condition that causes inflammation of the joint, and in 2011 it affected 27 million people. Unlike other conditions that cause joint pain, it does not affect your internal organs or other parts of your body. It is frequently found among older people, although children can have it too. Up until age 45, men are more likely to be diagnosed with osteoarthritis but afterward it is more common in women. Both women and African-Americans are more likely to have OA of the knee.

The older one is the greater the likelihood of having it. OA of the knee is found in 37 percent of people over 65. It is important to note that you do not get osteoarthritis from getting older.

The major risk factors for OA are: genetics (there are families who get OA very early, without the other risk factors), being overweight/obese (increasing risk with increasing weight), being inactive, and sustaining a significant injury. You may get OA with each one of these factors, but if you have several of these risk factors, then you are more likely to get OA earlier and more severely. At the same time, there are people who have OA who had not sustained an injury. The risk of getting OA is multifactorial, and none is absolute. Osteoarthritis is a condition that should be taken very seriously not only because if ignored it can limit your mobility but because it can impact your overall health.

A major study in England of 1,163 people over the age of 35 found that people with osteoarthritis of the hip or knee were more likely to die earlier from all causes than the general population.

CAUSES AND PREVENTION

Most of the time osteoarthritis is due to the progressive wearing down of joints caused by an inherited tendency to have weak cartilage, excess weight, lack of physical activity, or joint injury. For some people, the work they do may cause repetitive stress to the joints, and they have to find a way to do their work in a different way. For others, old injuries result in osteoarthritis later in life. People who were physically active when they were younger and had knee, hip, shoulder, hand, foot, or back injuries find that later in life they develop osteoarthritis in those joints they thought had healed.

Most osteoarthritis is found in the hands and knees. The hip is another area where you can have OA. Women are more likely to have osteoarthritis in their hands if their mother or grandmother also had it. This suggests that at least for osteoarthritis in the hands there may be some genetic factors that should be considered.

In order to prevent OA, there are three actions you can take. First, if you have excess weight, try to lose as much weight as you can. This is not about looks but about the mechanics of joints. Excess weight creates more pressure, which in turn increases the grinding of the bones that only worsens the joint over time. Every pound of extra overall weight equals the force of three pounds on the hip joint and four pounds on the knee joint. Second, make movement a part of your life. It is important to keep the joint as flexible as possible by doing stretching as well as strengthening exercises and to be as mobile as you can be. You need to talk to your health care provider about what types of exercises you should be able to do. Third, when you have pain or are injured, take care of your joint immediately. Pain is the way that your joints tell you to stop what you are doing. If you do not stop doing whatever is causing you pain, you will continue to damage yourself. The worse thing to do if you are involved in any sport is to try to "play through the pain." This may seem like the thing to do "for the team," but the negative consequences for you and your family can last the rest of your life.

Q *Do I have a problem?*
Sometimes you have a pain in your joint and you know that what you need to do is rest the joint for the pain to go away. At other times, if your joint feels stiff, you have pain, and the pain does not go away, it would be better to see your health care provider. According to NIAMS and arthritis experts the warning signs of osteoarthritis are:

- **Pain.** It is worse when using the joint and is relieved by rest. Pain can also change with damp, cold, rainy weather, making someone with arthritis feel like a weather forecaster who can predict when a storm is coming.
- **Stiffness.** After being in one position for a long time, the joint feels stiff. This includes sitting or getting out of bed. The stiffness is of short duration, lasting less than 30 minutes.
- **Swelling.** The joint that hurts is also swollen. The swelling is often due to bony overgrowth around the joints.
- **Sound.** When you move the joint, you hear the sound of bones grinding.

Osteoarthritis can cause the joint to deteriorate to the point where you become unable to move on your own because of the severe pain you experience. This is most likely to occur when you have osteoarthritis in your back (neck and spine), knees, and/ or hips. The inability to move exacerbates the situation because you are no longer able to engage in the physical activity that is essential for weight management and to maintain flexibility.

TREATMENT

There is no cure for osteoarthritis. Your health care provider will work with you to develop a treatment plan that will focus on making you comfortable and improving your activity level. This means that you will work to reduce pain, improve as much as possible the amount of movement of the joint which is pain free, and maintain a healthy weight to reduce the wear and tear on the joint. Each of these strategies is discussed below.

Pain

Limiting the motion of the joint that hurts may be the first thing you try. It turns out that movement and strengthening the muscles around your joint will make your joint feel better and can improve your pain. For your arthritis pain, your health care provider may recommend heat or cold be applied to the joint along with medication (see page 89). The medicine your health care provider recommends will take into account your history, other medicines you are taking, and the benefits and risks associated with each medicine. Make sure you talk with your health care provider about risks associated with pain medication to find the right approach for you, and make sure you consistently monitor the effects of the medicine. You may find that specific topical creams that you put on the joint help you. Find one that works for you and use it. In addition, your health care provider may suggest that you use a cane. A cane should be held in the hand opposite to the lower joint effected with OA. Your health care provider may recommend other things you can use to reduce the pain you have with movement (assistive devices). In some instances when the problem is in the knee a series of three to five injections to increase the lubrication in the knee may be suggested. According to the Agency for Healthcare Research and Quality (AHRQ), there is little evidence to support this procedure.

Range of motion

Your health care provider will tell you what type of exercises you should do. Your exercise program should include both stretching and strengthening. Keep in mind that even though your health care provider or physical therapist tells you to do something, you should stop if the pain is too great. Let him or her know that you have pain so that he or she can recommend a different exercise that will keep the joint flexible and not give you pain. It is also a good habit to put ice on the joint after you exercise.

Healthy weight
Your health care provider will work with you to support your efforts to have a healthier weight. Excess weight makes it more difficult for the underlying mechanics of the joint to function properly.

While OA of the knee is the most common condition, we have not made much progress in learning how to treat it. In April 2009 the AHRQ analyzed the evidence on the effectiveness and safety of three treatments for OA of the knee. They specifically looked at (1) use of specific supplements—glucosamine, chondroitin, or both; (2) injection of hyaluronan (viscosupplementation), a major component of the synovial fluid into the knee; and (3) arthroscopic surgery to clean the debris (bone bits) in the joint area. In each instance the treatment outcomes were usually compared to those of persons who received a placebo. In all three instances the conclusion was the same: given the available research "none of the treatments reviewed . . . were effective for the general population of people with knee osteoarthritis." In one study they found that for some people with moderate to severe OA glucosamine and chondroitin provided some relief of pain and that they were better able to move their knee, but these had no measurable effect on people with mild pain.

 What can I do?
If you are diagnosed with osteoarthritis, you will have to be more thoughtful about many aspects of your

life. Use the information provided in the 10-Point Program for Health and Wellness as your starting point.

Rheumatoid arthritis (RA)

I have been engaged in sports for as long as I can remember. Physical activity has been part of what I did throughout my entire life. I watch what I eat, and I have not gained weight. And now every time I move, my joints hurt. I have a constant ache, and I don't know what to do about it. It even hurts when I sit. —Alicia

Although it had been a long time since I had seen Eduardo, I did not expect to see him in a wheelchair. He looked at me and, with a sad smile, said, "You must be surprised to see me like this. I am too. You know I never knew I had rheumatoid arthritis. I just thought my aches and pains were from my old football injuries . . . something that would just happen because I was getting older. I thought I knew. I was wrong. I waited so long to see a doctor that by the time I did go and find out that I had rheumatoid arthritis, I had very few options." —Adolpho

Q *¿Qué pasa?*
Rheumatoid arthritis is an autoimmune disorder in which your body attacks your joints. When you have

RA, one of the things that happens is that your immune system produces an inflammatory response. This is how the immune system usually protects you from microbes that attack your body, but when you have RA there are no microbes. That is why you may find that your joints swell. Sometimes it may be the same joint, but sometimes it may be another joint. Over time the inflammation can dissolve the cartilage and bone, resulting in joint pain and deformity.

CAUSES AND PREVENTION

We do not know what causes RA. There is no cure. In many instances with medication, it is possible to completely control the disease and stop the joint destruction and deformity. Since we do not know the cause of RA, the focus of prevention is to reduce some of the known risk factors. We know that people who have family members with rheumatoid arthritis or who smoke are more likely to develop RA.

Q *Do I have a problem?*
We know that RA occurs more often in women than in men. Only your health care provider can tell you for sure if you have RA. He or she will ask you about your symptoms, complete a physical exam to assess what are the movements you can do without pain and what are the ones that cause discomfort, and may do other blood tests to rule out other conditions.

The warning signs of RA are:

- **Morning stiffness.** This lasts for many hours. This is in contrast to OA, where the morning stiffness lasts less than 30 minutes.

- **Swelling.** The joints are warm, often red and swollen.
- **Loss of joint mobility and strength,** such as not being able to make a fist or open a door.
- **Other organ involvement.**

RA can result in general tiredness, and the inflammation can affect your lungs, heart, and blood vessels, possibly resulting in a stroke, and can affect your skin, causing lumps to appear on your elbows or hands called rheumatoid nodules.

In some instances your health care provider may take x-rays. Unfortunately, x-rays are not as informative as they are for other conditions. Some people who have severe damage do not experience much pain and others with severe pain have x-rays that reveal only minimal damage. In the latter case, your health care provider may suggest another kind of imaging test.

TREATMENT

While there is no cure for RA, there is excellent treatment that can control the inflammation. Your health care provider will work with you to develop a treatment plan that is consistent with your abilities, resources, and obligations. Treatment will work to slow the progression of the condition, control pain, lessen deformity, and improve function.

- **Slowing the progression.** Disease-modifying anti-rheumatic drugs (DMARDs) are used to slow or stop the immune system from attacking the joints. If taken early, they can stop or slow further damage to the joint; they cannot repair joints that are already damaged. Drugs commonly used are methotrexate and the biologics such as anti-TNF medications (see pages 92–93).

- **Controlling pain.** Medication, creams, hypnosis, acupuncture, and other methods are used to decrease the pain that is experienced. Since pain is so very subjective, the approach has to be tailored to the individual. There is some early research that fish oil and gamma-linolenic acid may be beneficial.
- **Improving function.** Key components will include weight control as a means of reducing the impact on your joints and keeping your joints functioning well with strengthening and stretching exercises. It may be that your health care provider will suggest visiting an occupational or a physical therapist to show you safe exercises and joint protection activities, along with equipment such as splints that you may need to use in your home and work life so you reduce the likelihood of further injury.
- **Mood.** It is also important to be mindful of your mood. Recent studies suggest that nearly 40 percent of people who know they have rheumatoid arthritis seem to have symptoms of depression. This is especially true for people with more modest incomes. Depression should not just be ignored since it makes it harder for you to take care of yourself. This is particularly problematic when you have a condition like rheumatoid arthritis where you need to be actively involved in your own care as part of a lifelong strategy. Moreover, people who have depression who do not seek treatment are also more likely to have other health conditions.

Q *What can I do?*
Because RA is a chronic condition, it will be very important for you to see a health care professional early, since the sooner RA is treated, the less joint destruction occurs. This makes it especially important for you to follow the plan you develop with your health care provider, track all aspects of your health (see pages 112–15), maintain good and ongoing communication with all of your health care providers, and listen to your body. The 10-Point Program for Health and Wellness will reinforce all the positive steps you take to control your RA. You may want to add walnuts, flax, olive oil, beans, and cold-water fish to your diet. All of these are high in omega-3 fatty acids. Diets high in these fatty acids have been shown to reduce joint inflammation.

Lupus

Q *¿Qué pasa?*
This is an autoimmune disease that can attack your joints, skin, kidneys, heart, lungs, blood vessels, or brain. There are five major types of lupus.

1. **Systemic lupus erythematosus, or SLE.** This is the most common type of lupus. It typically affects many parts of your body.

2. **Discoid lupus erythematosus.** You get a skin rash that does not go away.

3. **Subacute cutaneous lupus erythematosus.** After you are in the sun, you get skin sores.

4. **Drug-induced lupus.** You have a side effect to a medication you are taking.

5. **Neonatal lupus.** This rare type of lupus affects newborns.

Some of the more common symptoms of lupus are: pain or swelling in your joints, muscle pain, a fever that has no known cause, red rashes (most often on the face), pain in your chest when you take a deep breath, you start to lose your hair, the color of the skin on your fingers or toes gets pale or purple, you become sensitive to the sun, you find that you have swelling in your legs or around your eyes, you get ulcers in your mouth, your glands seem to get swollen, and/or you feel very tired. There are other symptoms too, but all of them come and go with varying degrees of severity. When you have symptoms they are called flare-ups.

CAUSES AND PREVENTION

With the exception of a drug-induced form of lupus, there is no known cause. In all likelihood a combination of genetic, environmental, and biological factors may trigger lupus.

Q *Do I have a problem?*
This is a very difficult condition to diagnose or treat. It can take months or even years to get an accurate diagnosis. This condition occurs in both men and women, although nine out ten people with lupus are women. Hispanics and African-Americans are more likely to have lupus than non-Hispanic whites.

The most common symptoms are:

- **Skin.** A rash over your nose and cheeks that is sensitive to sun exposure is common. It is called a butterfly rash.
- **Hair loss.** Patches of hair loss can occur, leaving bald spots.
- **Chest pain.** Pain occurs when taking deep breaths.
- **Arthritis.** The joints can become swollen with morning stiffness.
- **Kidney.** Inflammation in the kidneys can result in swollen ankles.
- **General tiredness and increased body temperature.**

TREATMENT

Your health care provider will develop a treatment plan for you with three main goals: (1) to prevent flare-ups, (2) to treat episodes when they occur, and (3) to reduce damage to the affected areas. This will probably mean that you will take medicines, have to track your health on a regular basis, and pursue those activities that are consistent with your treatment plan. Pain management will be a part of your treatment plan as the joint pain with lupus can be very intense.

Q What can I do?
You need to supply your health care provider with the best information about your symptoms and any changes you experience. This means that you must not only be engaged in your health care but you must also be proactive. By working with your health care team, you will be able to maximize the benefit you get from your treatment plan.

◠ Other rheumatic conditions

There are many other rheumatic conditions. What follows is some information on the ones about which there is the most research available. They are generally difficult to diagnose and for most of them the cause is not known. It would be accurate to say that in most instances a combination of genetic and environmental factors play a significant role in the condition.

Ankylosing spondylitis (spinal arthritis)

My back was causing me a lot of pain, and I was referred by a friend to see the best orthopedist in town. He was the physician for a major sports team, and if anyone could help me I knew that he would help me. He examined me and said he would start treatment the following week for my spinal problems. I mentioned that I had had inflammation of my eyes years before and other symptoms. It did not seem to matter to him and for some reason that left me unsettled. Then a few days later I started to think about it and talked to some other physicians. When I saw a rheumatologist he listened carefully, did some further tests, and told me that I had ankylosing spondylitis. To this day I consider myself lucky to have found him and to have started the right kind of treatment early. —Nancy

Q *¿Qué pasa?*
Your back is in pain, and you do not seem to find any relief. This is probably caused by the stiffening of a joint (ankylos), specifically the vertebrae (spondylo) or nearby structures. Another defining characteristic is inflammation of the joints located where the spine joins the pelvis (sacroiliitis). The blood tests of people with ankylosing spondylitis are negative for the rheumatoid factor. Disorders with these characteristics are called seronegative spondyloarthropathies. Most people (80 percent) develop this condition before age 30 and only 5 percent develop it after age 45. It is also more common in men than in women.

CAUSES AND PREVENTION
The cause is unknown although there is some role for genetics. HLA-B27 is a gene that about 8 percent of Americans have. Among non-Hispanic whites the gene is found in more than 95 percent of people who have ankylosing spondylitis. The gene is not found as much in African-Americans and people from some Mediterranean backgrounds who have ankylosing spondylitis. Additionally, there are people who have the gene but do not develop ankylosing spondylitis. The two other genes of interest are ERAP1 (previously known as ARTS1) and IL23R.

Q *Do I have a problem?*
Your health care provider will take your medical history and do a physical exam. In this case x-rays are of limited value because they do not reveal the damage resulting from the disease until there is considerable deterioration. MRIs, although expensive, provide a good image of the soft tissue and bones.

Symptoms of ankylosing spondylitis are:

- **Back pain.** The back pain becomes worse with rest, causing morning stiffness and pain for more than 30 minutes and improves with exercise.
- **Heel pain.** Swelling and pain in the heel and stiffness of the tendons behind your heels can occur after rest.
- **Arthritis.** The hips, knees, ankles, and feet are most effected with pain, stiffness, and swelling.
- **Eyes.** One third of people with spinal arthritis develop painful eyes that become worse with light. This is called iritis.

TREATMENT

A treatment plan will be developed for you that includes appropriate medication.

Q *What can I do?*
Follow your treatment plan, stay active, and practice good posture. The latter is important because it gets you into the habit of using all the muscles that support your spine.

Complex regional pain syndrome (CRPS) (also called causalgia or reflex sympathetic dystrophy)

Q *¿Qué pasa?*
This is a nerve disorder of your central or peripheral nervous system. Half of the people who get this condition have been subjected to some kind of injury. There is intense pain in one of your arms, hands, legs, or feet that was injured. In CRPS I there is no underlying nerve injury, and in CRPS II there is underlying nerve injury. It is likely that the pain could have started in a finger that was injured and later spread to your entire arm.

CAUSES AND PREVENTION
The cause is unknown. Very little is known about this condition. It occurs in men and women, although it is most common among young women.

Q *Do I have a problem?*
Talk to your health care provider about all of your symptoms. The area where you have the pain might have significant changes in temperature (specifically it will be a different temperature than your other extremity), there may be changes in color (blotchy, purple, pale, or red), you might experience an intense burning sensation, and your skin can be extremely sensitive. You can have swelling and stiffness in

the affected joints, resulting in an inability to move that part of your body.

TREATMENT

Most of what your health care provider will do is focus on reducing pain through medication, physical therapy, and, as a last resort, nerve blocks. Nerve blocks can be achieved either through injection or surgery. It seems that rest makes the condition actually become worse.

Q *What can I do?*
Do the best you can to reduce your pain and discomfort. In some cases the symptoms go away on their own. Sometimes this relief is temporary, and in other cases it is permanent.

Dermatomyositis (inflammatory myopathies)

Q *¿Qué pasa?*
This is a condition that affects your muscles. You have inflammation of your muscles that does not go away and results in painless muscle weakness of your large muscles in your arms, legs, and body.

CAUSES AND PREVENTION

There is no known cause. Some people with lupus or other autoimmune diseases develop this condition.

Q *Do I have a problem?*
There is usually a skin rash before there is a flare-up. The rash looks patchy with purple or red areas, and develops on eyelids and on muscles used to extend or straighten joints, including knuckles, elbows, knees, and toes. Red rashes may also occur on the face, neck, shoulders, upper chest, back, and other locations, and there may be swelling in the affected areas. Sometimes there is a rash and no muscle pain. Some adults may lose weight, have a low-grade fever, or have problems with their lungs. Others find that they are sensitive to light, and that light makes the rash and their other symptoms get worse. Another symptom is the development of hard bumps under the skin or in the muscle that are actually calcium deposits called calcinosis. Your health care provider can check for increased muscle enzyme levels such as creatine kinase (CK) in your blood or take a piece of your muscle to make a diagnosis.

TREATMENT

Treatment includes a combination of anti-inflammatory medication, physical therapy, exercise, heat therapy (including microwave and ultrasound), orthotics and assistive devices, and rest. Treatment is usually successful. People with lung or heart disease do not respond as well to treatment.

Q *What can I do?*
There is little that you can do to prevent this condition. Following your treatment plan is the best option.

Fibromyalgia

Q *¿Qué pasa?*
This common syndrome causes pain and tenderness in different parts of the body and many other symptoms such as headaches and chest and back pain. It is not a disease because it has neither a specific cause or causes nor recognizable signs and symptoms. Fibromyalgia comes from the Latin term for fibrous tissue (*fibro*) and the Greek ones for muscle (*myo*) and pain (*algia*). This condition does not kill you, and it does not damage your muscles, joints, or internal organs.

CAUSES AND PREVENTION

The cause is unknown. It is believed to be triggered by traumatic events (physical or emotional). Women are more likely to have it than men. People with lupus, rheumatoid arthritis, or ankylosing spondylitis are at an increased risk of having fibromyalgia.

Q *Do I have a problem?*
There is no diagnostic test for fibromyalgia. It is very hard to diagnose this syndrome because the symptoms are common to many other conditions. Some of these include cognitive and memory problems (sometimes referred to as "fibro fog"), sleep disturbances, morning stiffness, headaches, irritable bowel syndrome, painful menstrual periods, numbness or tingling of the extremities, restless legs syndrome, temperature sensitivity, and sensitivity to loud noises or bright lights. You may have many areas of your body that are tender to touch, especially around your chest, neck, lower back, and

knees. Unfortunately, usually a person has to see many health care providers before they are properly diagnosed with this syndrome.

TREATMENT

Finding a health care provider who already treats people with fibromyalgia is a good place to begin. This is a condition that is very hard to treat and having a team of health professionals working with you is very helpful.

Q *What can I do?*
The 10-Point Program is a good start, but there are some specifics that should be highlighted. Make sure that you do all you can to get enough sleep. You also need to engage in a reasonable amount of physical activity. You should make as many changes at work as possible to accommodate your condition. Remember to eat for your health. Most of all, remain hopeful.

Gout

I woke up and thought I had an ingrown toenail. My big toe hurt so very, very much. I looked at it, and it looked normal but the pain was excruciating. I did not want to call my internist because it was only my toe that hurt. It seemed a waste of time and money to take off from work and go in for a visit just because of my big toe. But the pain was becoming increasingly worse, and I could barely walk. It felt like there were shards of glass in my toe. When I saw my internist he told me that because I had changed my diet so drastically by eliminating all carbs I had triggered what became my one and only gout attack. He prescribed some medicine and before long I was fine. And to think it all began with an extremely painful big toe. —Elena

Q ¿*Qué pasa?*
Purines are found in most foods. When you eat them, your body breaks them down into uric acid. Gout occurs when you have a build-up of uric acid. When your body processes the food you eat and the liquids you drink, it also leaves some substances that are not used and which are considered waste products. Uric acid is a waste product that is normally flushed out of your body in your urine. When you have gout, the uric acid builds up in your body in the form of crystals in some of your joints. Initially this build-up occurs in the big toe. Over time there can be build-up of these crystals in your insteps, ankles, heels, knees, wrists, fingers, and elbows. This accumulation of crystals is very, very painful. Gout is more common in men than in women.

CAUSES AND PREVENTION

We do not know what causes gout. We know that people with gout should avoid foods that are high in purines. Purines are found in our cells and in most foods. Some foods that have a high level of purines and therefore should be avoided are: asparagus, bacon, beef, bluefish, bouillon, cauliflower, chicken, chicken soup, codfish, crab, duck, goose, halibut, ham, kidney beans, lamb, lentils, lima beans, lobster, mushrooms, mutton, navy beans, oatmeal, oysters, peas, perch, pork, rabbit, salmon, shellfish, snapper, spinach, tripe, trout, tuna, turkey, veal, and venison. Some people also need to avoid all types of alcoholic drinks.

Q Do I have a problem?
You need to see your health care provider to know for sure. A very painful big toe is usually a symptom of gout. At other times it is difficult to diagnose since gout can resemble other conditions. Sometimes your health care provider may want to draw some fluid from the joint to see if there are uric acid crystals present. You can develop deposits of uric acid in your skin resulting in bumps that are called tophi.

TREATMENT

Most gout is treated with medication to lower the uric acid in your blood and make the tophi go away.

Q What can I do?
Take your medications regularly and drink lots of water as water helps remove uric acid. Avoid alcohol since that raises the uric acid level in your blood. Maintaining a healthy weight and a regular exercise program are also good. Eat nutritionally balanced meals because diets that are too low in carbohydrates can result in ketones that increase the uric acid in your blood.

Infectious arthritis

Q *¿Qué pasa?*
You were exposed to a microbe (bacteria, fungus, etc.) that entered your blood stream and this has caused a painful joint. You may also have a fever.

CAUSES AND PREVENTION

Since this is infectious, you usually have some idea of how you were exposed to the microbe.

Q *Do I have a problem?*
Infection in a joint causes severe pain in the joint, and you are likely to have a fever. It is important to go to your health care provider as soon as possible to get the right treatment. Your health care provider will take your history and do a physical exam. Additionally, he or she may use a needle to draw some fluid from the joint that is painful. In some cases this can reduce the pain and some of the fluid may be analyzed to determine the source of the infection. However, some bacteria that cause joint pain (gonorrhea, Lyme disease, and syphilis) are difficult to identify using this type of procedure.

TREATMENT

Your treatment will depend on the nature of your infection. You may be treated with an antibiotic, an antifungal, or an antiviral. Treatment must be quick because certain infections can destroy a joint in a very short time.

Q *What can I do?*
Take your antibiotics as soon as possible, and let your health care provider know how you are doing. It is likely that if you do not improve within 48 hours that a different medicine will be prescribed.

Polymyalgia rheumatica

Q *¿Qué pasa?*
This is a rheumatic disorder that causes muscle stiffness and pain in the neck, shoulders, and hips. Some people also have a fever, feel weak, and lose weight.

CAUSES AND PREVENTION

The cause is unknown. It is related to problems in the immune system. Genetic factors and some sort of infection trigger it. This condition is believed to be related to aging as it is rarely found in people younger than 50 years of age. Moreover, the number of people with the condition increases with age, with the highest number among 70- to 80-year-olds. Non-Hispanic white women are at increased risk for this condition. For people older than 50, the rate is 700 out of every 100,000 developing polymyalgia rheumatica. Polymyalgia rheumatica can be associated with inflammation of the blood vessels in the head that causes headaches, scalp tenderness, and, in rare instances, blindness.

Q *Do I have a problem?*
There is no single test to determine if this is what you have. A key finding is evidence of increased blood sed-

imentation rate, or ESR. People with this condition rarely have blood test results that are positive for rheumatoid factor. Specific lab tests may be recommended to rule out other conditions.

TREATMENT

Anti-inflammatory medications are very successful, and it can take one to several years to decrease the symptoms. The medication most often used is prednisone.

Q *What can I do?*
Follow your treatment plan to get some quick relief.

Psoriatic arthritis (PsA)

Q *¿Qué pasa?*
This condition occurs when someone who has psoriasis also develops arthritis. It is not rheumatoid arthritis with psoriasis. There are five types of psoriatic arthritis: symmetric (same joint on both sides of the body); asymmetric (one or many joints); distal interphalangeal predominant, or DIP (the joint closest to your fingernail or toenail); spondylitis (spinal column); and arthritis mutilans (small joints of hands and feet and sometimes neck or lower back). We know that non-Hispanic whites are more likely than African-Americans or Asians to develop PsA. These data are similar to what we know about psoriasis. At present there is no data about Hispanics.

Causes and Prevention

The cause is unknown. Most people are diagnosed with psoriasis between the ages of 15 and 35. Only 6 to 42 percent of people with psoriasis develop PsA. PsA often is diagnosed about 10 years after the initial diagnosis of psoriasis. Scientists are hoping to discover genetic markers on their road to find a cure.

Q *Do I have a problem?*
You need to talk to your health care provider. Since you are already treating your psoriasis, you will let your health care provider know of any painful joints, stiffness in your joints that lasts more than 30 minutes in the morning, limited range of motion, or tenderness that you experience. Early diagnosis helps to prevent further deterioration of the joint.

Treatment

Although there is no cure, treatment will reduce pain and decrease the amount of damage to the joint. Medications used to treat rheumatoid arthritis are used in PsA, such as DMARDs and biologics (see pages 92–93).

Q *What can I do?*
Learn to pace yourself. The extreme fatigue that is sometimes part of PsA may require that you rethink your daily schedule. You need to rest, but you also need to stay active. Talk to your health care provider about what you can do.

Scleroderma

Q ¿*Qué pasa?*
This umbrella term is used for the range of conditions that occur when there is overproduction of collagen. Collagen is a family of proteins that helps to build skin, tendon, bone, and other connective tissues. Too much collagen is a problem because it affects your connective tissue. Connective tissue is what supports your skin and internal organs. The severity of this condition ranges from affecting only the skin to damaging your internal organs. There are two major classes of conditions: localized (affects parts of the body) and systemic (affects the whole body).

CAUSES AND PREVENTION

We do not know the cause of this autoimmune disease. What is certain is that you can neither catch it from someone nor pass it from one person to another. Research with twins has further shown that it is not an inherited disease. Compared to men, women 30 to 55 years old are 7 to 12 times more likely than men to be diagnosed with scleroderma.

Q *Do I have a problem?*
Initially you may notice that your fingers and toes become white and painful if exposed to cold. This is called Raynaud's phenomenon. In addition, your skin becomes thickened and tight, limiting your mobility. Your medical history and physical exam will be important in helping your health care provider diagnose your condition. During your physical exam your health care provider will look for changes

in your skin's appearance and texture, including swollen fingers and hands and tight skin around the hands, face, mouth, or elsewhere; hard bumps that are calcium deposits developing under the skin; changes in the tiny blood vessels (capillaries) at the base of the fingernails; and patches of skin that have become thick. If it seems that you have scleroderma, your blood may be tested to see if it has some of the antibodies that are found in people who have scleroderma. These antibodies are antitopoisomerase-1 or Anti-Scl-70 antibodies and anticentromere antibodies. But none of these tests is definitive, and you may have to undergo other procedures.

TREATMENT

Scleroderma requires treatment by a variety of health professionals. It is important to have one person serve as the point person for coordination of your treatment. Depending on what is happening with your condition, there will be great variability in how to proceed.

What can I do?
The focus of all your efforts is to reduce pain, limit damage, and have the fullest life possible.

Juvenile idiopathic arthritis (JIA) (previously known as juvenile rheumatoid arthritis)

Q *¿Qué pasa?*
There are approximately 294,000 children under the age of 18 who have arthritis. JIA includes at least seven conditions:

1. **Systemic arthritis.** The child has joint pain, a fever, and a rash. About 25 percent of children with systemic arthritis have severe destructive joint disease.

2. **Oligoarthritis.** During the first six months, no more than four joints are affected. Additionally, the child may have inflammation of the eye (uveitis).

3. **Polyarthritis with negative rheumatoid factor.** During the first six months, five or more joints are affected.

4. **Polyarthritis with positive rheumatoid factor.** During the first six months, five or more joints are affected. This is a more destructive joint disease. The positive factor must occur in two blood tests taken at least three months apart.

5. **Enthesitis-related arthritis, or ERA.** This condition affects 11 to 16 percent of children with JIA. This autoimmune disease involves inflammation of

the area where tendons and ligaments attach to a bone. Children may also have an inflammation in their eye. This is more common in boys. While initially it may affect the hip, knee, and foot, the pain can later extend to the lower back. Children will say they have more discomfort when they are at rest than when they are active. The blood tests of children with this condition are positive for the human leukocyte antigen (HLA) B27 gene.

6. **Psoriatic arthritis.** Children have the joint pain of arthritis and a skin rash that is diagnosed as psoriasis. They may also have inflammation of the eye.

7. **Other (undifferentiated).** This catchall category includes all instances that are not listed above but where there is joint inflammation and pain that lasts at least six weeks. It is also used when a child has more than one of the conditions included under JIA.

CAUSES AND PREVENTION

The cause of all of these conditions is unknown. While there is no cure, there is treatment. The statistics show 70 to 400 of every 100,000 children have JIA.

Q *Do I have a problem?*
Only your health care provider can diagnose JIA. It is important to have a diagnosis as early as possible to reduce the damage that occurs when the condition is left untreated. The most common joint involved is the knee. Children

commonly do not complain of pain and just stop using the joint involved. They will appear stiff and often limp after sleeping in the morning or after naps.

TREATMENT

There are very few pediatric rheumatologists. Consequently, most children are seen by health care providers who treat adults. The treatment of JIA has been shown to be very effective, and the earlier the treatment is started, the better the chance the child will have normal growth and development. The medications used are similar to those used for rheumatoid arthritis and have been shown to work well in children. Because some of the treatments have just been introduced in the past 15 years, the long-term side effects are not known, but to date no major side effects have been found.

Q *What can I do?*
If you know someone with JIA, the goal is to help them get through their daily activities with minimal pain and discomfort. The goal is to make the necessary accommodations that will keep them engaged with others and involved in their evolving health care.

⌇ Understanding treatment

For most rheumatoid conditions there is no cure, and as a result you and your health care provider will develop a treatment plan. At a minimum your treatment plan will include weight management (to decrease stress on your joints), movement (to help mobility and help maintain a healthy weight), and medication and other procedures (to reduce pain and to stop or slow the progression of the condition).

This section is to help you better understand the various treatment methods that may be used to manage your condition. Often what you may know about the treatment of arthritis from talking to others may not be what is considered the best option for you. For example, while a supplement may be the answer for one person, someone with rheumatoid arthritis may experience greater benefit from a DMARD, while a third person with lupus uses both. There is great variability in the medicines that are available for each person.

Moreover, much of the treatment involves managing pain. This makes it even more imperative to tailor what you do to your experience and the results you achieve. In this section there is a presentation of the available options for treatment so that you can fully appreciate what are the limitations and possibilities. They are presented in alphabetical order.

Clinical trials

Q *What is this?*

Sometimes when people want to try a new treatment because they are looking for better outcomes they think about enrolling in a clinical trial. Clinical trials are essential to understanding how to improve our health. A clinical trial is the only method that we have to know whether some intervention (medicine, procedure, etc.) actually does what it claims to do. It is a research study that is done with people who meet specific criteria. By the time there is a clinical trial, the medicine or procedure has usually been tested in animals.

Criteria for including or excluding someone from a clinical trial may include factors such as a person's age, gender, the type and extent of a disease or condition, previous treatment history, and other medical conditions. These criteria are based on what questions are being studied in the clinical trial. Sometimes a clinical trial only includes people who have a specific condition and at other times it only includes people who do not have any conditions.

Some clinical trials are called interventional studies because individual participants in the study are assigned by the researcher to a specific treatment or other intervention to document the impact of the intervention. In this type of study, the specific aspects of an individual's health are monitored to see what happens as a result of each of the interventions. The analysis focuses on the outcomes that are measured.

Another kind of clinical trial is an observational study in which the participants are observed on specific factors, and the outcomes are measured by the researcher. Observational studies also have specific criteria that participants must meet to be included in the study.

A clinical trial can focus on one of the following aspects of a condition: prevention, diagnosis or screening, treatment (experimental treatments, new combinations of drugs, or new approaches to surgery or radiation therapy), or quality of life (supportive care). Each trial also has phases that have different purposes and try to answer specific questions about safety and effectiveness. Each of the phases is described below:

- **Phase I.** 20–80 people receive an experimental drug or treatment for the first time to evaluate its safety, determine a safe dosage range, and identify side effects.
- **Phase II.** 100–300 people receive an experimental study drug or treatment to see if it is effective and to further evaluate its safety.
- **Phase III.** Includes 1,000–3,000 people to confirm that the experimental drug or treatment is effective, monitor side effects, compare it to commonly used treatments, and collect information that will allow the experimental drug or treatment to be used safely.
- **Phase IV.** After the experimental drug or treatment is used in the broader population, there is ongoing monitoring of the risks, benefits, and optimal use associated with the drug or procedure.

Q *How does it work?*
In interventional clinical trials, some people receive the new treatment and others do not. Who gets what

type of treatment is determined based on the study protocol. In most instances, one of the groups will be given either a placebo treatment or the current standard of care to see if the new medicine or procedure is measurably better than what is already done. A placebo may be a pill, liquid, or powder that has no active substances in it or an intervention that is known to have no treatment value. It is very important to understand this because sometimes what appears to have an impact is due to a placebo effect. A placebo effect is a change, occurring after an intervention, that is not the result of any special property of the intervention and in fact reflects more the expectation of the participant. Some researchers believe that the placebo effect may reflect the strength of the mind-body connection that some people have.

If you decide to be part of a clinical trial, you should expect the process to include time to address all aspects of informed consent. The decision to participate in a clinical trial is very important and one that requires a clear understanding of the study that is being proposed, as well as the risks and benefits of being a part of the clinical trial. The research team has the obligation and responsibility to provide you with an informed consent document that includes details about the purpose, duration, and required procedures that are part of the study, as well as the risks and benefits of participation. You should also receive the contact information for the staff involved in the study. This document should be provided in the language that you feel most comfortable reading.

Read the document carefully, and when you do not understand something, you should ask questions. You need to understand what will be your financial and other responsibilities. If you agree to participate, you can sign the document with the understanding that it is not a contract. This means that at any time in the future you can withdraw from the study.

Q *What can I expect?*

The process for the clinical trial is determined by the type of study that is being undertaken and the phase of the study. Most clinical trial teams include a researcher, physician, and other types of health care professionals who are responsible for monitoring the health of the participants and implementing the study. Some clinical trials may require additional tests and visits. The team will work to keep you informed about any new developments or information that you may need.

Medicines

Q *What is this?*

There are many types of medicines, prescription and those available without a prescription (over-the-counter, or OTC), that are used depending on the condition that is causing your arthritis. Some of the broad categories of medicines are discussed below.

Q *How does it work?*

Each medicine works in a different way. Newer medicines are developed to have fewer negative side effects and to target new factors that are related to a given condition.

ANALGESICS (PAINKILLERS)

These are medicines that you take to relieve pain. The major types are:

1. Paracetamol (acetaminophen)

2. NSAID (non-steroidal anti-inflammatory drug, such as ibuprofen or Advil®)

3. Nonselective NSAIDs (csNSAIDs)

4. COX-2 inhibitors (selective cyclooxygenase-2 inhibitors or coxibs). These include rofecoxib and celecoxib.

5. Opioids and morphine-related medications (morphine, codeine, oxycodone, hydrocodone, dihydromorphine, pethidine)

6. Creams or ointments (topical analgesics)

In 2006 one out of every five people in the United States received a prescription for an analgesic. These painkillers are very popular and represent a major source of relief for persons who have a rheumatoid condition. Each medicine works in a slightly different way to reduce pain.

Paracetamol (acetaminophen), opiates, and morphine-related medications work on the brain. These medicines alter the chemistry in your brain so that you do not feel pain. They work well to reduce mild pain and have few side effects.

Aspirin makes it difficult for the platelets in our blood to clump and make a blood clot. According to the AHRQ, aspirin should be considered in its own category because it is different from other NSAIDs.

NSAIDs work equally well for moderate to severe pain. At the same time they increase the chance of gastrointestinal bleeding and are especially difficult for people over 75. People who have had instances of gastrointestinal bleeding should avoid NSAIDs; instead they should consider taking acetaminophen.

Most NSAIDs work by reducing the body's capacity to produce an enzyme (cyclooxygenase, or COX). Having less of this enzyme in the body reduces the inflammation and pain because it decreases the production of a related molecule (prostaglandin). Further research discovered that there were at least two types of the COX enzyme. COX-2 inhibitors only impact on COX-2. While these reduced the side effects that could develop with NSAIDs, there were concerns that they increased the risk for heart conditions and stroke. Vioxx® was in this class, but is no longer available in the United States. The future of COX-2 inhibitors is still unfolding.

While many of the NSAIDs are available without a prescription, COX-2 inhibitors are available only by prescription. Keep in mind that NSAIDs need to be taken very thoughtfully and after discussion with your health care provider. In some cases NSAIDs have caused stomach problems and other side effects. The Food and Drug Administration (FDA) issued a specific warning for people who have heart problems who use NSAIDs for many years. The FDA stated that they had an increased risk of having a heart attack or stroke.

Some people cannot take medicines and instead rely on creams and ointments to relieve the pain in their joints. In these cases, the cream or ointment is rubbed or applied to the painful joints and works in a variety of ways. Some of these ointments work by irritating the surface of the skin. It is believed that the irritation takes the focus of the brain away from the painful joint. These counterirritants include menthol, oil of wintergreen, eucalyptus oil, or camphor, and are found in over-the-counter products such as Eucalytamint and Icy Hot®. Other creams (Aspercreme®, BenGay®, and many others) have salicylates that were believed to block the chemicals that cause pain. An analysis by the AHRQ indicated that products with salicylates had no effect on the pain from osteoarthritis. Products with capsaicin, which occurs naturally in cayenne peppers, is also said to relieve chronic pain for people with osteoarthritis. Even though this works for some, about half of all people who use a capsaicin-based cream also experience a burning sensation that seems to go away after a while. Some people who use a topical cream or ointment also take pills to feel better.

BIOLOGICS (BIOLOGIC RESPONSE MODIFIERS)

These relatively new medicines are genetically engineered. The word *biologic* refers to the fact that these relatively new medicines are made from proteins that come from living cells. They are neither made from chemicals that occur naturally nor are they produced in a laboratory. Most people with RA (about two-thirds) and those with PsA, ankylosing spondylitis, and JIA are able to stop the progression of the disease as long as they are getting a biologic. While they work by not letting the immune system attack your body (immunosuppressant), this also makes the individual more vulnerable to infections. You usually take these by injection or intravenously over several hours (infusion). Some of the most commonly prescribed are etanercept, adalimumab, infliximab, abatacept, and rituximab. In April 2011 the FDA approved the use of tocilizumab (Actemra®) for systemic juvenile idiopathic arthritis.

CORTICOSTEROIDS

These medicines stop the immune system from attacking the joints (immunosuppressant) and reduce the inflammation. They can be taken as pills, lotions, or by injection. While short-term use has some side effects (increased appetite, dramatic and uncharacteristic mood swings, swelling, facial hair), long-term use has more serious side effects (high blood pressure, cataracts, high blood glucose, infections). The most common corticosteroids are prednisone, cortisone, solumedrol, and hydrocortisone.

DISEASE-MODIFYING ANTI-RHEUMATIC DRUGS (DMARDs)

These medicines are used to treat conditions such as rheumatoid arthritis and ankylosing spondylitis. They work by slowing or stopping the immune system from attacking the joints (immunosuppressant), which unfortunately also leaves the person more likely to get an infection. DMARDs include methotrexate, hydroxychloroquine, sulfasalazine, and leflunomide. Methotrexate is one of the older DMARDs, and as a result there is a lot of information about how to best use it. Early diagnosis is essential to prevent further damage to the joints. DMARDs are not easily grouped into a class of medicines and you may experience success with one DMARD but not another. Sometimes adding a DMARD makes the other medicine (including another DMARD) work better. DMARDs are very powerful, and many have side effects that you need to discuss with your health care provider. Some are listed below:

Generic Name	Brand Name
Pills	
hydroxychloroquine	Plaquenil®
leflunomide	Arava®
methotrexate	Rheumatrex®
	Trexall®
sulfasalazine	Azulfidine®
	Sulfazine®
Injections	
adalimumab	Humira®
anakinra	Kineret®
certolizumab pegol	Cimzia®
etanercept	Enbrel®
golimumab	Simponi®
Given Intravenously (Infusion)	
abatacept	Orencia®
belimumab	Benlysta®
infliximab	Remicade®
rituximab	Rituxan®
tocilizumab	Actemra®

Q *What can I expect?*
Medication is a key component of the management of arthritis. You will have to maintain good communication with your health care provider. In that way, he or she can make the adjustments that may be required to make your medi-

cines do the best job possible. The combination of medication you will take will be tailored to your specific situation.

We know that there is variability in the effectiveness of analgesic medication based on age and other factors. In a study of older adults (average age 80 and 85 percent were women) with arthritis, use of opioids was more likely to cause death than use of NSAIDs. Additionally, there was an increased risk for fractures in persons who used opioids. These findings were based on analyzing the records of 12,840 Medicare beneficiaries in Pennsylvania and New Jersey.

Pain and pain management

Q What is this?

One of the major symptoms of any condition that causes inflammation of the joints is pain. A key part of ongoing treatment will involve pain management. There are a variety of medicines that are used to decrease pain. Your health care provider will work with you to find which is the most effective for you.

You should be aware that pain and pain management is a huge area for health fraud. Too many people are willing to try anything to get rid of pain. As a result sometimes the only person who feels better is the one who feels good about selling fraudulent products or procedures.

Talk to your health care provider about your options. Biofeedback, massage, progressive relaxation, acupuncture, and other alternative procedures and techniques have given some benefit to some people with pain. A major study funded by the

National Institute of Arthritis and Musculoskeletal and Skin Diseases (NIAMS) and the National Center for Complementary and Alternative Medicine (NCCAM) concluded that acupuncture "relieves pain and improves function in knee osteoarthritis, and it serves as an effective complement to standard care." The value of acupuncture for people with RA is uncertain and needs more research. According to the NCCAM, part of the National Institutes of Health, some mind-body techniques, specifically relaxation, imagery, tai chi, and biofeedback, may help improve symptoms associated with RA. For some people there are positive effects when these therapies are added to a treatment plan that consists of primarily conventional medical treatments.

Q *How does it work?*
Medicines and other procedures work by either masking the pain or decreasing the inflammation that causes the pain.

Q *What can I expect?*
Your health care provider will ask you to rate your pain and to keep a record of the pain you experience and what you do to get relief. Being accurate is very important since this information is essential for developing a plan that will make you comfortable and keep you active.

The future in pain management looks brighter. The NIH Pain Consortium is looking to develop tools for individualized pain management, documenting emerging therapies, and trying to make available to consumers the newest scientific findings on pain management.

Supplements, herbs, and teas

Q *What is this?*
According to the FDA a dietary supplement is a product taken by mouth that contains a "dietary ingredient" that you consume in addition to your regular meals. The "dietary ingredients" in these products may include: vitamins, minerals, herbs or other botanicals, amino acids, and substances such as enzymes, organ tissues, glandulars, and metabolites. Dietary supplements can also be extracts or concentrates, and may be found in many forms, such as tablets, capsules, softgels, gelcaps, liquids, or powders. They can also be in other forms, such as a bar, but if they are, information on their label must not represent the product as a conventional food or a sole item of a meal or diet.

It is important to know that supplements are regulated under the broad umbrella of "food" and not "drugs." This means that the manufacturer of a dietary supplement or dietary ingredient is responsible for ensuring that it is safe before it is sold but does not have to prove that it is either safe or effective for the intended use. Specifically, the FDA does not have to "approve" dietary supplements for safety or effectiveness before they reach the consumer. That is why it is illegal for a product sold as a dietary supplement to promote on its label or in labeling that it is a treatment, prevention, or cure for a specific disease or condition.

You also need to know that what is actually in a supplement can vary since there is no regulation to ensure that you get the same substance in the same amount in each pill. This variance in purity makes comparisons difficult.

There are very few clinical studies with supplements. The Glucosamine/chondroitin Arthritis Intervention Trial (GAIT) was the first large-scale clinical trial in the United States to test the effects of glucosamine hydrochloride (glucosamine) and sodium chondroitin sulfate (chondroitin sulfate) for the treatment of knee osteoarthritis. In this study funded by the NIAMS and NCCAM, participants received either:

Glucosamine alone: 1,500 mg daily, given as 500 mg three times a day;
Chondroitin sulfate alone: 1,200 mg daily, given as 400 mg three times a day;
Glucosamine plus chondroitin sulfate combined: 1,500 mg and 1,200 mg daily;
Celecoxib (COX-2 inhibitor): 200 mg daily; or
Placebo

The findings were mixed. Overall, there were no significant differences between the other treatments tested and the placebo. However, for a small subset of participants with moderate-to-severe pain, glucosamine combined with chondroitin sulfate provided statistically significant pain relief compared with the placebo. For participants in the mild pain subset, glucosamine and chondroitin sulfate either taken alone or in combination did not provide significant pain relief.

Another part of the study looked at whether these dietary supplements could diminish structural damage from osteoarthritis of the knee. The results were perplexing because in the ancillary study, interested GAIT patients were offered the opportunity to continue their original study treatment for an additional 18 months, for a total of 2 years. At the end of the ancillary study, the team had gathered data on 581 knees. After assessing the x-ray data, the researchers concluded that glucos-amine and chondroitin sulfate, together or alone, appeared to fare no better than the placebo in slowing loss of cartilage in os-teoarthritis of the knee. Interpreting the study results was com-plicated, however, because participants taking the placebo had a smaller loss of cartilage, or joint space width, than predicted.

There is much to learn, but at the very least we need to be aware of what these supplements are and to stay alert for any new research that is forthcoming.

There are supplements that on their label imply that they are a cure or treatment for arthritis. It is best to focus on the ones for which there is some information. Keep in mind that for any of these, there is limited information available and a lack of high-quality research that focuses on dose, duration of treat-ment, or long-term effects. Some of the supplements of interest are discussed below:

Boswellia (*Boswellia serrata, Boswellia carterii*, also known as frankincense)
Lab and animal studies suggest that the resin of this plant pro-duces a substance that has anti-inflammatory effects and that it also affects the immune system.

Chondroitin (chondroitin sulfate)
This is a complex carbohydrate that helps cartilage retain water.

Curcumin
Extracts of turmeric (*Curcuma longa*) contain the chemical cur-cumin. In studies with animals it was found to protect joints from inflammation and damage. There is ongoing research to understand the anti-inflammatory effects of curcumin and RA.

Fish oil

Fish oil contains high amounts of omega-3 fatty acids. Your body may be able to use omega-3s in supplements to make substances that reduce inflammation. Some fish high in omega-3s are herring, mackerel, salmon, and tuna. According to the NCCAM, the evidence from clinical trials on RA is encouraging. You need to tell your health care provider if you are taking any supplements with fish oil since high doses may interact with certain medicines, including blood thinners and drugs used for high blood pressure. Additionally, some products made from fish liver oil (for example, cod liver oil) can contain dangerously high amounts of vitamins A and D.

Gamma-linolenic acid (GLA)

GLA is an omega-6 fatty acid found in the oils of some plant seeds, including evening primrose (*Oenothera biennis*), borage (*Borago officinalis*), and black currant (*Ribes nigrum*). Your body may be able to convert GLA into substances that reduce inflammation and relieve symptoms such as joint pain, stiffness, and tenderness.

Ginger (*Zingiber officinale*)

In the lab, it has been shown that ginger contains compounds that are known to be anti-inflammatory.

Glucosamine

This is an amino sugar produced by the body and found around cartilage and other connective tissue. When people take these supplements, they experience varying degrees of relief ranging from no relief to some relief.

Green tea

Some of the compounds in green tea may be helpful with RA and OA. It seems that the active ingredients in green tea may inhibit the chemicals and enzymes that damage cartilage.

Thunder god vine (*Tripterygium wilfordii*)

Extracts are prepared from only the skinned root of this herb because the other parts of the plant are highly toxic. This extract has been used in China for centuries and is known to cause severe side effects such as diarrhea, upset stomach, hair loss, headache, and skin rash. It is generally not available in the United States. According to the best available data from the NIAMS, thunder god vine may fight inflammation and suppress the immune system, but the negative consequences of long-term use outweigh benefits.

Vitamins C, D, and E or beta-carotene

It may be that the rate of joint deterioration of OA is slowed when people take larger doses of these vitamins. Ask your health care provider about the dosage you should take because large doses of vitamin D can be harmful.

Q How does it work?
We usually do not know because the manufacturers of dietary supplements are not regulated by the FDA the same way as manufacturers of medicines. Specifically, this means that dietary supplements may interact in unknown ways with medications or other supplements or may have unknown side effects. Since the labeling requirements are different from the requirements for labeling medicines, some supplements may contain potentially harmful ingredients not listed on the

label. Moreover, since clinical data are not required most supplements have not been tested in pregnant women, nursing mothers, or children. Also there are no standards or oversight for manufacturing and one pill may vary greatly from another. Finally, the reporting of side effects from supplements leaves much to be desired.

Q *What can I expect?*

The important fact is that if you have RA or some other autoimmune disorder, it is not a good idea to replace your conventional medicine with an unproven complementary and alternative medicine (CAM) therapy regardless of how convincing the video, ad, presentation, or individual may be. The FDA reminds consumers to be alert when they see the words *natural* and *herbal.* Too often all these words do is convey a false sense of wholesomeness or an implication that these foodlike substances will have milder, if any, side effects.

You must tell your health care provider about all the supplements and other substances you take. Coumadin (a prescription medicine), ginkgo biloba (an herbal supplement), aspirin (an OTC drug), and vitamin E (a vitamin supplement) can each thin the blood. According to the FDA taking any of these products together can increase the potential for internal bleeding. St. John's Wort, another popular supplement, reduces the effectiveness of certain drugs used to treat HIV, heart disease, depression, seizures, and certain cancers, as well as the effectiveness of some oral contraceptives.

Surgery

My mother had to have her knees replaced so I was not surprised that I had to have my knees replaced. My surgeon wanted me to do both knees at the same time but I thought one would be enough. It has taken a long time to heal. —Laura

Q *What is this?*
In some cases the damage in the joint requires surgery. Surgery is rarely recommended if your arthritis is due to an autoimmune condition. You need to exercise care and caution before embarking on surgery since it is not the first choice of treatment (medication, pain management, and lifestyle changes are first). Moreover, recovery planning is critical.

Most of the time surgery is done in what is referred to as a "minimally invasive surgical procedure." In this type of procedure, the surgeon uses a special scope with a miniature camera (arthroscope) that allows him or her to look inside the joint and use other tiny tools to make the repairs. This means that small instruments are inserted through two small incisions. One incision is to allow for the entry of the tools necessary for the repair and the other incision is for the arthroscope. The surgeon can see the joint as the images from the camera are shown on a television monitor. Surgery may be done to remove loose pieces of material that are in the joint (arthroscopy), move the bones (osteotomy), or smooth out the ridges on the bone (joint resurfacing). Sometimes open surgery is required, where the surgeon makes a larger incision and uses regular instruments. In more severe, advanced cases, the joint may be replaced. The most recent research says that arthroscopic surgery of the knee is helpful for conditions excluding osteoarthritis.

For women, replacement of the hip or knee is often more complicated than for men. Keep in mind that replacement of a joint is major surgery that requires many months of rehabilitation.

The recent FDA hip implant recalls show it is vital to ask lots of questions, including if the surgeon receives payment from the implant manufacturer, the track record of implant performance, and whether the risk of a newer device with less real-life data is warranted.

Q *How does it work?*
It is intended to repair the damaged joint.

Q *What can I expect?*
Arthroscopic surgery will require less time to recover and heal than open surgery. If you need to have your knee or hip replaced, it is likely that you will be in the hospital for several days and will need help at home to get things done for several weeks. Additionally, you will have to rearrange your work schedule to ensure that you attend regular sessions for physical therapy and rehabilitation.

One of the most promising areas of research involves "patching" a joint so that new cartilage will grow. This research is using stem cells found in a person's fat tissue to form a scaffolding at the joint that will be stimulated with biochemicals and grow new cartilage.

Part Three

RESOURCES AND TOOLS TO HELP YOU TAKE CONTROL

Vital Information and Best Sources

If you have questions about arthritis, please call the National Hispanic Family Health Help Line at 1-866-783-2645 or 1-866-SU-FAMILIA. Health promotion advisors are available to answer your questions in English and Spanish and to help you find local services. You can call Monday through Friday, from 9 A.M. to 6 P.M. ET.

You can also contact the Arthritis Foundation by calling 1-800-283-7800, where customer service representatives are available to answer your questions in English and Spanish. This is a free, 24-hour hotline available to anyone.

Best Noncommercial Websites

While there are many sites that offer to treat arthritis or relieve pain with a product or a process, the websites listed below are dedicated to providing you the best information available and will not sell any personal information you provide. Additionally, none of these sites allows advertising or product endorsements.

Agency for Healthcare Research and Quality (AHRQ)
www.effectivehealthcare.ahrq.gov
The mission of AHRQ is to improve the quality, safety, efficiency, and effectiveness of health care for all Americans. As one of the agencies within the Department of Health and Human Services, the AHRQ supports research that helps people make more informed decisions and improves the quality of health care services. The AHRQ was formerly known as the Agency for Health Care Policy and Research.

ARTHRITIS FOUNDATION
www.arthritis.org

The mission of the Arthritis Foundation is to improve lives through leadership in the prevention, control, and cure of arthritis and related diseases. As the largest private, not-for-profit contributor to arthritis research in the world, the Arthritis Foundation is the leading health organization addressing the needs of the millions of people at risk for and living with arthritis in the United States.

CENTERS FOR DISEASE CONTROL AND PREVENTION (CDC)
www.cdc.gov

The CDC's mission is to collaborate to create the expertise, information, and tools that people and communities need to protect their health—through health promotion; prevention of disease, injury, and disability; and preparedness for new health threats.

CLINICAL TRIALS
clinicaltrials.gov

ClinicalTrials.gov is where you can find out about all federally and privately supported clinical trials conducted in the United States and around the world. ClinicalTrials.gov gives you information about a trial's purpose, who may participate, locations, and phone numbers for more details.

NATIONAL ALLIANCE FOR HISPANIC HEALTH
hispanichealth.org

The mission of the Alliance is to improve the health and well-being of Hispanics and work with others to secure health for all.

NATIONAL CENTER FOR COMPLEMENTARY AND
ALTERNATIVE MEDICINE (NCCAM)
  nccam.nih.gov
The mission of the NCCAM, part of the National Institutes of
Health, is to define, through rigorous scientific investigation,
the usefulness and safety of complementary and alternative
medicine interventions and their roles in improving health
and health care.

NATIONAL INSTITUTE OF ARTHRITIS AND MUSCULOSKELETAL AND
SKIN DISEASES (NIAMS)
  www.niams.nih.gov
The mission of the NIAMS, part of the National Institutes of
Health, is to support research into the causes, treatment, and
prevention of arthritis and musculoskeletal and skin diseases;
the training of basic and clinical scientists to carry out this
research; and the dissemination of information on research
progress in these diseases.

NATIONAL LIBRARY OF MEDICINE (NLM): MEDLINEPLUS
  www.nlm.nih.gov
The NLM, part of the National Institutes of Health, is the
world's largest medical library. The Library collects materials
and provides information and research services in all areas of
biomedicine and health care.

QUESTIONS TO ASK YOUR HEALTH CARE PROVIDER

About your diagnosis
- *What type of arthritis do I have?*
- *Will I get better?*
- *Are there things I should avoid doing?*
- *Should I see a rheumatologist?*
- *What can I do to reduce the pain in my joints?*
- *Should I put ice or heat on my joints when they hurt?*
- *Should I change what I eat?*

About your medicines
- *What are the medicines I should take?*
- *How do I take them?*
- *Are there any side effects?*
- *Will the arthritis medications interact with the medications I am already taking?*
- *When will the medicine start working?*
- *Should I take any supplements?*
- *Are there supplements or teas I should avoid?*

About your treatment plan
- *What exercises can I do?*
- *What do I do if it hurts too much when I exercise?*
- *Do I need to see a physical therapist?*
- *Would a cane help me with my walking?*

QUESTIONS YOUR HEALTH CARE PROVIDER WILL ASK YOU

According to the NIAMS, to get the best diagnosis you need to be prepared to give your health care provider the most accurate answers possible to the following questions:

- *Is the pain in one or more joints?*
- *When does the pain occur?*
- *How long does the pain last?*
- *When did you first notice the pain?*
- *What were you doing when you first noticed the pain?*
- *Does activity make the pain better or worse?*
- *Have you had any illnesses or accidents that may account for the pain?*
- *Are you experiencing any other symptoms besides pain?*
- *Is there a family history of arthritis or other rheumatic disease?*
- *What medicine(s) are you taking?*
- *Have you had any recent infections?*
- *Do you have any allergies or are you allergic to any medicines?*

VISITS TO MY HEALTH CARE PROVIDER

Date _____ Why I went _____

Whom I saw _____

Special tests _____

Diagnosis _____

Referred elsewhere _____

Medicines prescribed _____

What else did the health care provider do/say? _____

_____

_____

Date _____ Why I went _____

Whom I saw _____

Special tests _____

Diagnosis _____

Referred elsewhere _____

Medicines prescribed _____

What else did the health care provider do/say? _____

_____

_____

My medicines, vitamins, supplements, teas, and other things I take

Name _____ Cost _____
Purpose _____
Size/Amount _____ Color _____ Shape _____
Date prescribed _____ By _____
How much do I take? _____ When? _____
Things to avoid _____
Side effects/Other comments _____
_____

Name _____ Cost _____
Purpose _____
Size/Amount _____ Color _____ Shape _____
Date prescribed _____ By _____
How much do I take? _____ When? _____
Things to avoid _____
Side effects/Other comments _____
_____

Name _____ Cost _____
Purpose _____
Size/Amount _____ Color _____ Shape _____
Date prescribed _____ By _____
How much do I take? _____ When? _____
Things to avoid _____
Side effects/Other comments _____
_____

TOOLS TO TRACK MOOD, SLEEP, MEDICATION, AND PHYSICAL ACTIVITY

Tracking What I Do

"What I Am Doing" gives you a way to keep track of your mood, how healthy you are eating, social interactions, medication(s), sleep, and exercise. If you regularly write down what you are doing in these areas, you will be able to give your health care provider timely and valuable information that can help to fine-tune your treatment plan. You can also use this chart to see what factors change how your body feels and what is your overall mood from day to day. It is good to be able to identify what is helpful and what is damaging in your life.

Use the scale below for the first three items, and for the other items fill in the information as indicated.

1 = extremely negative
2 = moderately negative
3 = slightly negative
4 = neutral

5 = slightly positive
6 = moderately positive
7 = extremely positive

Mood: *How did you feel most of the day?*
Food: *How would you describe your overall food choices?*
Social: *How do you feel about your interactions with others throughout the day?*
All Meds: *Did you take all of your medicines? The answer here is yes or no.*
Sleep: *How many hours did you sleep last night?*
Exercise: *How many minutes of exercise did you do?*
Notes: *Add any information that you feel is important about the day.*

WHAT I AM DOING

(Scale of 1 = extremely negative to 7 = extremely positive)

Date	Mood (1–7)	Food (1–7)	Social (1–7)	All Meds (Yes/No)	Sleep (Hours)	Exercise (Minutes)	Notes

⌒ **Acknowledgments**

There are many people who make the *Buena Salud®* series possible. Esther Margolis, Heidi Sachner, Keith Hollaman, and Harry Burton provided incredible encouragement. The board, staff, and members of the National Alliance for Hispanic Health and the Health Foundation for the Americas also nurtured the series. Adolph P. Falcón, Senior Vice President of the Alliance, committed his heart and brains to making this series a reality. The translations were based on the collaborative efforts of Susana Bellido Cummings and Rosamaria Graziani. Their deep commitment and understanding of the *Buena Salud®* series were essential to the Spanish editions.

Dr. John Klippel, President and CEO of the Arthritis Foundation, encouraged me to write this book and dedicated the time to write the foreword. He is a champion for many and leads the movement to address arthritis in all communities. As CEO he has been a friend and an inspiration. Dr. Patience White, Vice President for Public Health for the Arthritis Foundation, reviewed this manuscript and shared her decades of wisdom to ensure that the science was at the cutting edge and reflected her clinical experience. Her gentle, firm manner is a joy for all who work with her as well as to her many grateful patients.

The personal support that I need to write comes from my life sisters and brothers, as well as exceptional individuals who are part of my life: Kevin Adams, Carolyn Curiel, Msgr. Duffy, Adolph P. Falcón, Polly Gault, Paula Gomez, Ileana Herrell, Thomas Pheasant, Bob Presbie, Sheila Raviv, Carolina Reyes,

ACKNOWLEDGMENTS

Esther Sciammarella, Amanda Spivey, Cynthia A. Telles, and Elizabeth Valdez.

My relationship with Margaret Heckler spans nearly three decades, throughout which she has shared her extensive knowledge, her belief in the greater good, her deep faith, and the importance of faith in everyone's lives. My memories and experiences with my extraordinary mother, Lucy Delgado, my cousin Deborah Helvarg, and my friend Henrietta Villaescusa are also part of everything that I am and all that I do. And most of all, on a daily basis the love and support of my husband, Mark, and my daughter, Elizabeth, have been the source of much joy and laughter in my life.

∽ Index

ABOUT THE AUTHOR

JANE L. DELGADO, Ph.D., M.S., author of *The Latina Guide to Health:* Consejos *and Caring Answers* and the *Buena Salud®* Guides, is President and Chief Executive Officer of the National Alliance for Hispanic Health ("the Alliance"), the nation's largest organization of health and human service providers to Hispanics. She was recognized by *Ladies' Home Journal* as one of the "Ladies We Love" in 2010 and by WebMD as one of its four Health Heroes of 2008 for her dedication and resilience in advocacy. Among many other awards and honors, in 2007 *People en Español* named her to the 100 Most Influential Hispanics.

A practicing clinical psychologist, Dr. Delgado joined the Alliance in 1985 after serving in the Immediate Office of the Secretary of the U.S. Department of Health and Human Services (DHHS), where she became a key force in the development of the landmark "Report of the Secretary's Task Force on Black and Minority Health."

At the Alliance, Dr. Delgado oversees the national staff as well as field operations throughout the United States and Puerto Rico. She serves on the National Biodefense Science Board. She is also a trustee of the Kresge Foundation, Lovelace Respiratory Research Institute, and the Northern Virginia Health Foundation, and serves on the National Board of Mrs. Rosalyn Carter's Task Force on Mental Health.

Dr. Delgado received her M.A. in psychology from New York University in 1975. In 1981 she was awarded a Ph.D. in clinical psychology from SUNY Stony Brook and an M.S. in urban and policy sciences from the W. Averell Harriman School of Urban and Policy Sciences. She lives in Washington, D.C., with her husband, Mark, and daughter, Elizabeth.

Founded in 1973, the **National Alliance for Hispanic Health** is the foremost science-based source of information and trusted advocate for the health of Hispanics. The Alliance represents local community agencies serving more than 15 million people each year, and national organizations serving more than 100 million people, making a daily difference in the lives of Hispanic communities and families.

The **Health Foundation for the Americas** (HFA) supports the work and mission of the National Alliance for Hispanic Health. Every year the HFA supports programs to improve health for all by helping secure clean air to breathe, clean water to drink, safe places to play, and healthy food to eat. The HFA and the Alliance help those without health care gain access to free and low-cost services where they live and improve the quality of health care. The programs put new health technology to work in communities, provide millions of dollars in science and health career scholarships, and conduct the research and advocacy that is transforming health.

You can be a part of this extraordinary mission of health and well-being. To learn more about the Alliance or the HFA, visit www.hispanichealth.org or www.healthyamericas.org.

The author donates all royalties from the Spanish editions of her books to the Health Foundation for the Americas (HFA).

Titles by Jane L. Delgado

Written specifically for the growing U.S. Hispanic population by Jane L. Delgado, Ph.D., M.S., the President and CEO of the National Alliance for Hispanic Health, the *Buena Salud*® Guides present the best in science and health advice, available in both English- and Spanish-language editions.

The *Buena Salud*® Guide to Overcoming Depression and Enjoying Life
Foreword by Former First Lady Rosalynn Carter, Founder, Carter Center Mental Health Program

Highlighted by real-life stories, this authoritative, accessible guide answers the most asked questions about depression, debunks common myths, and offers readers information they can trust on treating and managing this condition.

The book addresses: how to overcome cultural barriers to recognizing and seeking help for depression, including *machismo* and *aguantando* (enduring); the relationship between depression and chronic conditions such as diabetes, heart disease, and arthritis; medication, therapy options, genetics, and alternative treatments; lifestyle changes to help overcome depression; the social and physical differences in how men and women deal with depression; advice on choosing a psychotherapist; and a section covering treatment and other topics.

Paperback • 128 pages • ISBN: 978-1-55704-972-8 • $9.95

Also available in Spanish:
La guía de *Buena Salud*® para superar la depresión y disfrutar la vida (978-1-55704-974-2)

The *Buena Salud*® Guide for a Healthy Heart
Introduction by Jack Lewin, M.D., CEO, American College of Cardiology

Opening with a personal story from Dr. Delgado about her mother's experience with heart disease, this invaluable guide details everything readers need to know about the leading cause of death for all men and women in the United States.

The book explains: how the heart works; how heart problems develop and what can be done to avoid them; achievable lifestyle changes to maintain heart health; and features a section with commonly used heart terms and diagnostic tests and procedures.

Paperback • 128 pages • ISBN: 978-1-55704-943-8 • $9.95

Also available in Spanish:
La guía de *Buena Salud*® para un corazón sano (978-1-55704-944-5)

The *Buena Salud*® Guide to Diabetes and Your Life
Introduction by Larry Hausner, CEO, America Diabetes Association

Featuring the stories of people and families living with diabetes—a condition that has touched the lives of most Hispanic families—this concise guide explains everything readers need to know, including the important fact that diabetes is not inevitable.

The book discusses: the factors that contribute to developing diabetes and how to prevent it; the types and evolving definition of diabetes; how the endocrine and immune systems function; the impact of the environment on diabetes; treatment options, including medication and realistic changes in lifestyle and diet; and features a section with terms used to discuss diabetes.

Paperback • 128 pages • ISBN: 978-1-55704-941-4 • $9.95

Also available in Spanish:
La guía de *Buena Salud*® sobre la diabetes y tu vida (978-1-55704-942-1)

The Latina Guide to Health: *Consejos* and Caring Answers
Foreword by Antonia Novello, M.D., M.P.H., Dr. P.H.,
    Former U.S. Surgeon General

Featuring cutting-edge medical information and advice for all Hispanic women, Dr. Delgado offers practical information on the health issues women face, separates myths from facts, and answers questions about what to do. She discusses arthritis, cervical cancer, depression, and other important topics in a quick-reference health section.

Paperback • 240 pages • ISBN: 978-1-55704-854-7 • $15.95

Also available in Spanish:
La guía de salud: Consejos y respuestas para la mujer latina
    (978-1-55704-855-4)